COURGETTI

Delicious and easy recipes
for your spiralizer

JACQUELINE WHITEHART

PEPIK BOOKS

Pepik Books

York

www.courgettirecipes.com

Text © Jacqueline Whitehart 2016

Jacqueline Whitehart asserts her moral right to be

identified as the author of this work.

A catalogue record for this book is

available from the British Library.

ISBN: 978-0-9955318-0-2

All rights reserved. No parts of this publication may be reproduced, stored in a retrieval system or transmitted, in any form or by any means, electronic, mechanical, photocopying, recording or otherwise, without the prior permission of the publishers.

This book features weight-loss techniques which may not be suitable for everyone. You should always consult with a qualified medical practitioner before starting any weight-loss programme, or if you have any concerns about your health. This book is not tailored to individual requirements or needs and its contents are solely for general information purposes. It should not be taken as professional or medical advice or diagnosis. The activities detailed in this book should not be used as a substitute for any treatment or medication prescribed or recommended to you by a medical practitioner. The author and the publishers do not accept any responsibility for any adverse effects that may occur as a result of the use of the suggestions or information herein. If you feel that you are experiencing adverse effects after embarking on any weight-loss programme, including the type described in this book, it is imperative that you seek medical advice. Results may vary from individual to individual.

CONTENTS

INTRODUCTION

If you haven't tried 'Courgetti' you're in for a treat. Courgetti or Courgette Spaghetti can be made and served in less time than it takes to make conventional pasta. All you need is a spiralizer or even just a vegetable peeler. You can turn the humble and (dare I say it) boring courgette into the perfect healthy meal in minutes.

Learn how to make the perfect Courgetti

Discover what other vegetables to spiralize

Get help with finding the best spiralizer for you

Over 80 recipes including spaghetti, noodles and cucumber noodle salads. Whether you go for a traditional Italian pasta dish, an amazing stir-fry or a huge salad with cucumber noodles, you'll find flavoursome and satisfying dinners from every corner of the world.

REDUCING CALORIES AND CUTTING OUT WHEAT

Have you ever looked at your tummy after a big bowl of pasta? I have and I don't recommend it! You can clearly see that your stomach has expanded and is more rotund with the pasta. It will take a good night's sleep for it to go down. If you are in any way intolerant to wheat or suffer from digestive problems this can be even more pronounced. It is the sauce that we love rather than the taste of the pasta itself. So why not cut out the traditional pasta and replace it with something equally delicious but with a fraction of the calories and no wheat and no carbs?

It sounds too good to be true... but it's not. Once you've got the spiralizer and the easy technique sorted then it becomes second nature and you can get rid of the pasta once and for all.

LOW CARBS AND GOOD CARBS

I truly believe that a real balanced diet means cutting back on carbs so that they no longer dominate your diet. A healthy balance is simply good carbs, filling protein and healthy fats. Replacing conventional pasta with courgetti is a really simple way to change the balance of your meal. Courgette spaghetti contains no carbs and a small amount of healthy fat in the form of olive oil. Then it's up to you what you add to make a balanced meal. The majority of recipes here add protein in the form of meat, fish or dairy. You'll also find loads of recipes with slower digestion carbs such as lentils and beans. These good carbs make the meal more filling and keep you sustained for longer.

Although every recipe is calorie counted for your convenience, you'll find that when you eat a courgetti meal it's a lot lower calorie than its pasta equivalent. In essence, you've already made the swap to a healthier meal.

A low carb dinner, for which courgette spaghetti is the perfect base, is a great step towards healthy and sustainable weight-loss. You'll feel full without heaviness.

VEGETARIAN AND VEGAN

About half the recipes in this book are vegetarian. I love lentils and beans and as they add both protein and good carbs they are the perfect accompaniment to courgette spaghetti. Although not all the vegetarian meals here are vegan, you'll often find they can be easily adapted. For example, by not adding the sprinkling of parmesan cheese. Additionally, you'll find lots of the spicy and noodle dishes are 100% vegan.

CHOOSING THE RIGHT SPIRALIZER

If you don't know where to start then making the right purchase can seem a little daunting. There are many many different kinds of spiralizers out there, all claiming to be the best. The range of features and prices is huge.

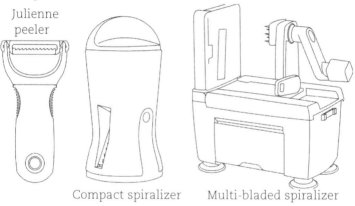

Julienne peeler

Compact spiralizer   Multi-bladed spiralizer

The good news is you really don't need to spend a fortune. A julienne peeler (that's a y-shaped peeler with teeth) costs about £5 and a simple spiralizer from approximately £10. More advanced spiralizers, usually signified by a turning handle, cost from £25 upwards. In my opinion all of these will work really well and hand-powered (as opposed to electric) is actually more practical in this case.

My criteria for choosing a spiralizer are as follows:

1   **Ease of use**

Does it work? Does it require a lot of effort and/or technique? Does it clog easily?

2   **Quality**

Are the blades sharp? Is it robust enough to stand up to regular usage? Are there bits that can break off?

3   **Price**

Is it good value for money? Would I recommend it to my friends?

4   **Safety**

All spiralizers have sharp teeth like blades. How far are the blades from my fingers during normal use? Would I let my kids use it? Am I likely to have to touch the blades to unclog or clean the device?

5   **Washability**

Will it go in the dishwasher? How do I clean the blades? Do I need to take it apart to wash it?

6   **Size and footprint**

Can it be stored in a drawer? Or does it require a cupboard or worktop space?

I have tried and tested all three of the main types of spiralizer. These are (1) A julienne peeler, (2) A compact spiralizer and (3) A multi-bladed spiralizer with a turning handle. A compact spiralizer has a cone at one end and you put your vegetable in and turn the vegetable, just as you would a pencil in a sharpener. A multi-bladed spiralizer sits on your work surface and you feed the vegetable in while turning a handle.

I will not be naming the brands of the spiralizers as I do not wish to endorse any one in particular. For the tests I have chosen the big brands and top sellers in each category. Scores are out of 10.

	Julienne peeler	Compact spiralizer	Multi-bladed spiralizer
Ease of use	8	9	8
Quality	7	7	6
Price	10	8	6
Safety	2	7	9
Washability	10	8	4
Size and footprint	10	9	6
	8/10	**9/10**	**6/10**
	If you're confident that you won't chop off your fingers then this is the perfect gadget. So simple and so cheap. Even goes in the dishwasher!	The best all-rounder. Works well. Nice and solid. Small. Easy to clean.	A bit too fiddly and big. Works better than the others when set up. But I fear it would languish in the cupboard of doom!

All the spiralizers were easy to use when set up, although I had to spend more time preparing the multi-bladed spiralizer for use. All were relatively robust. Although I worried about losing/breaking parts of the multi-bladed spiralizer.

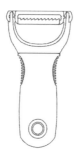

The **julienne peeler** can't be beaten on price, washability (it's the only one that goes in the dishwasher) or size but those blades are lethal and your fingers are only millimetres away during use. Would I let my kids use a julienne peeler? Definitely not.

The **multi-bladed spiralizer** was the best in so many ways – except in just actually producing courgette spaghetti reliably and fast. It felt as if it is too gadgety and I have no use for its additional blades and features. It's like the food processor, destined to live at the back of the

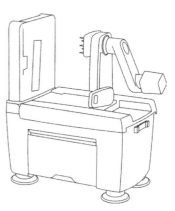

cupboard with the extra blades lost before first use.

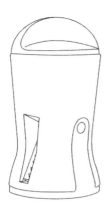

So the winner has to be the **compact spiralizer**. Solid, not particularly exciting, but gets the job done for a good price. When purchasing, make sure you choose one that comes with a cleaning brush. These are invaluable for cleaning out the little clogged bits of courgette from those spiky blades.

HOW TO MAKE THE PERFECT COURGETTE SPAGHETTI

IT'S AS EASY AS 1-2-3.

1   Spiralize or julienne your courgette
2   Blot on kitchen paper
3   Fry in a small teaspoon of oil for 2-4 minutes

PREPARATION

Choose your courgette. For one person I would choose a large straight courgette. When you spiralize your courgette, you'll find that you get masses and masses of spaghetti but the spaghetti reduces in volume by more than 50% when you cook it. So go large. You don't want a sad half full bowl of courgette spaghetti. If in doubt, go for 2 smaller courgettes. I've never had to leave any yet!

- One large courgette has 36 calories
- One medium courgette has 27 calories
- One small courgette has 19 calories
- A small teaspoon of oil contains 27 calories

Start with a large washed courgette. If you prefer you can peel the courgette at this stage but leaving the skin on adds colour and texture to the finished dish.

If you are spiralizing, trim the courgette at one end. If you are julienne peeling leave the ends on so that you can hold the end as you peel.

SPIRALIZING WITH A COMPACT SPIRALIZER

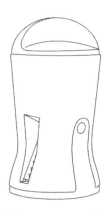

Place the trimmed end of the courgette in the fat end of the spiralizer and twist like you would a pencil in a sharpener. With a compact spiralizer you hold the spiralizer still with one hand and turn the courgette with the other. Press firmly and turn clockwise. Courgette spaghetti just pours out the side. The top of the courgette is soon sharpened to look just like a pencil.

When you reach the end of the courgette you can attach the cap to the nobbly end of the courgette and push the courgette further in to get more spaghetti and reduce wastage.

SPIRALIZING WITH A MULTI-BLADED SPIRALIZER WITH A TURNING HANDLE

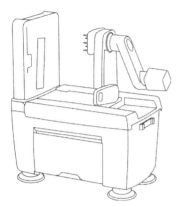

On a spiralizer with a handle you fit the courgette or other vegetable firmly onto adjustable spikes on the spiralizer. If your spiralizer has a stand make sure it is positioned securely on your worktop with suckers if available.

Choose the right blade for courgette spaghetti. As courgette does reduce in volume when cooked, I find the fatter or noodle blade is better as the spaghetti is less likely to break up when cooking. Fitting the courgette well onto the spikes is the key task to get right. Make sure it is fitted firmly and centrally. If the end of your courgette is not flat, you may find trimming the courgette so it fits snugly on the spikes is the best solution.

Start turning the handle slowly. It is a slow turn with a slight push towards the blades. Depending on your model, at the start you may also want to gently guide the courgette towards the blades with your other hand. Keep your fingers as far from the blade as possible. Place your kitchen paper where the spaghetti falls out of the spiralizer so it is ready to blot.

USING A JULIENNE PEELER

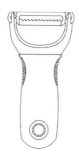 Start with one large washed courgette. Run the peeler down the full length of the courgette. Repeat on the same side making long pieces of courgette until you reach the seeds in the centre. Make a quarter turn in the courgette and begin again. Go all round the courgette until you have an oblong strip of seeds which can be discarded. Be careful as you near the end of the courgette as the julienne peeler is sharp and you could easily cut your finger.

NO SPIRALIZER OR JULIENNE PEELER? NO PROBLEM

Don't be dispirited if you don't have the right tool. You can still get started with courgette spaghetti and see if it works for you using a standard vegetable peeler. Using a normal peeler gives you wider thin strips of 'pasta'; you could call it tagliatelle. It cooks in exactly the same way as courgette spaghetti and still goes beautifully with a sauce.

To prepare courgette tagliatelle, start with one large peeled courgette. A peeled courgette is better for this dish as otherwise you get some strips of 'pasta' that are just skin. Then run the peeler down the full length of the courgette. Repeat on the same side making long pieces of courgette until you reach the seeds in the centre. Make a quarter turn in the courgette and begin again. Go all round the courgette until you have an oblong strip of seeds which can be discarded. Then proceed to blotting and cooking as normal.

BLOTTING ON KITCHEN PAPER

If your courgette spaghetti has ever come out as a spongy messy unappetizing blob then this is probably where you are going wrong. If you do not blot your courgette before cooking it will steam instead of stir-fry. Seriously, this is where everybody seems to go wrong and is the most important tip I can give you.

"Don't forget to blot!"

It's so simple. Lay out 2 pieces of kitchen paper on your work surface. When you spiralize, let the courgette fall straight onto the paper. When you've done spiralizing, spread the courgette roughly around the paper. Get two more sheets of kitchen paper and press down over the top. Leave it as a 'sandwich' for just 2 minutes and a huge amount of water will be absorbed into the kitchen paper and the courgette spaghetti is ready to cook.

"Just 2 minutes wrapped in kitchen paper before cooking is all you need."

Of course leaving it a bit longer than 2 minutes is fine too. When the courgette spaghetti is all wrapped up, then you can start preparing the pan and heating the oil ready for cooking.

COOKING TECHNIQUE

Cooking the courgette spaghetti couldn't be easier. The pan just needs to be sizzling hot before you add the courgette and you'll avoid soggy spaghetti.

- Heat a small teaspoon of olive oil in a large wide frying pan on a high heat. Heat for approximately one minute. If you wish, check that the pan is hot enough by dropping in one piece of spaghetti to see if it sizzles. Make sure you put the spaghetti in before the oil starts to smoke.

- Drop all the courgette into the pan and use a wooden spoon to push it round so it is evenly spread across the base of the pan.

- Season generously with salt and pepper.

- Don't over stir. Leave for about a minute after adding to the pan and then toss gently every minute until cooked.

- The perfect courgette spaghetti takes 2-4 minutes and should be soft with a few burnt edges.

Top tip

Add extra flavour with garlic or chilli oil for courgette spaghetti. The oil from a tub of sun-dried tomatoes is also delicious in a tomato dish. Alternatively, try walnut or sesame oil when making stir-fry or noodles.

SPIRALIZING OTHER VEGETABLES

The best and easiest vegetables to spiralize are courgettes, cucumber and carrots. Most other root vegetables, such as parsnip and butternut squash also spiralize well.

Also possible, but not quite so easy are the denser 'layered' vegetables such as onion and cabbage. Fruits with a crisp flesh, like apples, also spiralize well. Any vegetable which is in anyway soft or hollow will not spiralize.

Courgette

Trim top and bottom. Wash (or peel if preferred) and spiralize.

Cucumber

Trim top and bottom. Peel. Spiralize. Can be halved lengthways if necessary.

Carrot and parsnip

Peel and cut off top. Spiralize.

Butternut squash

Trim base so it stands flat. Peel downwards to base. Split vertically and hollow out seeds in the centre. Divide lengthways into quarters or eighths before spiralizing.

Onion

Trim top and bottom and peel. Quarter, then spiralize.

Cabbage

Remove loose outer layers and wash. Split into quarters or eighths depending on size. Cut out the central core before spiralizing.

Apple

Peel. Quarter and core. Spiralize.

RECIPES

A QUICK WORD ABOUT CALORIE COUNTING

All the recipes here have been individually calorie counted. The calories listed under the recipe title are the calories per portion. Although all efforts have been made to make these calorie counts as accurate as possible, they can only be approximate as the exact calorie count of each ingredient will vary depending on the size of vegetable used or the fat content of meats and dairy.

Where the recipe says serve over courgette spaghetti, the calories for courgette spaghetti are not included in the recipe. For these recipes you should add on 63 calories for 1 large courgette (36 cals) cooked in a small teaspoon of olive oil (27 cals).

For example, Quickest Ever Tomato Sauce contains 60 calories. If served over courgette spaghetti it would contain 123 calories. If you then added a teaspoon of freshly grated parmesan with 21 calories the entire meal would still only contain 144 calories.

10 QUICK SAUCES

If you want a delicious meal in minutes, then these flavour-packed sauces can all be cooked in 5 to 15 minutes.

. . .

Quickest Ever Tomato Sauce

Chicken Pesto

Sun-dried Tomato Pasta Sauce

Greek-style Courgette Spaghetti

Mexican Beans and Cheese

Leek and Mushroom

Hot Chilli Prawns

Garlicky Lemon Spaghetti

Creamy Spicy Sausage

Herby Cheese and Chickpea

Quickest Ever Tomato Sauce

60 calories

Want to get your courgette spaghetti to table in under 5 minutes, together with a delicious sauce? Well this is the recipe for you.

Serves 1 • Ready in 5 minutes

1 tsp garlic oil
....
1 tsp tomato purée
....
2 fresh tomatoes, finely diced
....
2 slices jalapeno peppers (from a jar),
finely chopped
....

- Heat the garlic oil in a small pan and fry the tomato purée until just sizzling. Add the tomatoes and jalapenos and cook lightly for 3-4 minutes until the tomatoes have broken down into a sauce.

- Serve immediately over just cooked courgette spaghetti. Top with a little grated parmesan if desired.

Chicken Pesto

231 calories

So easy but so good....

Serves 1 • Ready in 15 minutes

1 tsp olive oil

1 x 150g skinless chicken breast, diced

2 tbsp water

1 heaped tsp good quality pesto

- Heat the oil in a shallow frying pan over a medium heat. Fry the chicken for 10-12 minutes, stirring occasionally, until cooked through and crispy. Remove from the heat and add the water. Stir to deglaze the pan, then add the pesto and stir through.

- Serve over freshly cooked courgette spaghetti. Add a sprinkling of fresh parmesan if desired.

Sun-dried Tomato Pasta Sauce

105 calories

No cooking required – just blitz and you're done! For added flavour, stir-fry your courgette spaghetti in the sun-dried tomato oil.

Serves 2 • Ready in 5 minutes

50g sun-dried tomatoes in oil
Handful (about 10) fresh basil leaves
2 cloves garlic, peeled
20g grated parmesan
1 tbsp water

- Simply place the sun-dried tomatoes, basil leaves, garlic and parmesan in a blender and blitz until roughly chopped and mixed. Add the water if necessary to help it mix.

- Stir into the cooked courgette spaghetti and serve with a little fresh basil and parmesan sprinkled over.

Greek-style Courgette Spaghetti

248 calories

This rich and flavoursome sauce takes only minutes
to cook.

Serves 1 • Ready in 5 minutes

1 spring onion, trimmed and sliced
1 tsp tomato puree
1 heaped tsp harissa paste
50g ready-to-eat lentils
3 tbsp water
30g goats' cheese, cubed or crumbled
4 large black olives

- In a small pan, dry fry the spring onion, tomato puree and harissa paste together for 1 minute.
- Add the lentils and water and simmer for 2 further minutes. Finally add the goats' cheese and melt in for as long as you want. Personally I like the warm gooey messy version – but each to their own!
- Stir through the courgette spaghetti and arrange the olives over the top.

Mexican Beans and Cheese

209 calories

These beans add a bit of pizzazz to your spaghetti.
As the flavour improves with time, you can leave some
spare for another day; it will keep well in the fridge for
2–3 days.

Serves 2 • Ready in 5 mins

1 x 400g tin kidney beans, rinsed and drained
1 tsp mild chilli powder
½ tsp ground cumin
1 tsp dried oregano
2 medium tomatoes, roughly chopped
40g Cheddar cheese, grated
Salt and freshly ground black pepper

- Tip the drained beans into a shallow bowl and roughly mash with the back of a fork. Sprinkle over the chilli powder, cumin, oregano and a generous sprinkling of salt and pepper. Mix together until thoroughly combined. Stir through the tomatoes.

- Add a generous serving of the bean mixture to the just cooked courgette spaghetti in the pan. Stir through and cook until warmed.

- Sprinkle over the grated cheese before serving and place under the grill if you like your cheese all deliciously melty.

Leek and Mushroom

245 calories

The flavours here are deep and autumnal. Will warm you up on a cold day.

Serves 1 • Ready in 15 minutes

1 tbsp olive oil
3 medium leeks, cut into 1cm rings
150g chestnut mushrooms, washed and sliced
juice ½ lemon
freshly ground salt and pepper
sprinkling (10g) parmesan cheese

- Heat the oil in a wide lidded frying pan or non-stick saucepan. Add in the leeks and fry on a medium heat for 5 minutes, stirring occasionally until the leeks have some brown bits. Add the mushrooms and continue to fry for a further 2 minutes.

- Then add 2 tablespoons water, turn up the heat and put the lid on the pan. Cook for 5 minutes, then remove the lid. If there is any liquid remaining cook with the lid off until the water has boiled off.

- Remove from the heat and stir in the lemon juice. Stir through courgette spaghetti and top with salt, pepper and parmesan cheese.

Hot Chilli Prawns

190 calories

This quick and easy sauce is a perfect accompaniment to Courgette Spaghetti.

Serves 1 • Ready in 5 minutes

1 tsp olive oil
1 clove garlic, peeled and crushed
1 tsp tomato purée
30g jalapeño peppers from a jar, drained and chopped
2 tomatoes, chopped
100g cooked and peeled king prawns
Freshly ground black pepper
10g Parmesan, finely grated

- Heat the oil in a frying pan over a medium heat and fry the garlic and tomato purée for a minute before adding the jalapeños and chopped tomatoes. Fry for 2–3 minutes, until the tomatoes start to soften.

- Add the prawns and warm through for a couple of minutes. Season generously with black pepper and serve immediately, sprinkled with the grated Parmesan.

Garlicky Lemon Spaghetti

81 calories

This is a great easy dish that can be knocked up in 5 minutes flat.

Serves 1 • Ready in 5 minutes

1 clove garlic, peeled and crushed
Zest of half a lemon
10g butter
Juice of half a lemon
Salt and freshly ground black pepper

- Cook the courgette spaghetti as normal but add the crushed garlic and lemon zest to the pan as you fry it.
- When the spaghetti has cooked, remove from the heat but leave in the pan. Add the butter and lemon juice and stir until the butter has melted. Season with salt and pepper to taste.

Creamy Spicy Sausage

334 calories

A quick and flavoursome dinner using store cupboard and frozen ingredients. I love using Polish smoked kabanos in this dish but any smoked sausage would work well.

Serves 2 • Ready in 12 minutes

100g smoked pork sausage, thinly sliced
....
150g frozen Mediterranean vegetables
....
1 tbsp wholegrain mustard
....
50ml double cream
....
Salt and freshly ground black pepper
....

- Place a large non-stick frying pan over a medium heat. Fry the sausage without any oil for 3–4 minutes until just turning brown. Remove with a slotted spoon and set aside, leaving the fat that's come out of the sausages in the pan.

- Add the vegetables to the frying pan, season with salt and pepper and fry over a high heat until tender, about 5 minutes. Reduce the heat to low and add two tablespoons of water. Stir in the mustard and sausage. Finally add the cream and heat through for 2 minutes until warm. Serve immediately.

Herby Cheese and Chickpea

200 calories

This is a filling and tasty meal in minutes. Just add courgette spaghetti.

Serves 1 • Ready in 4 minutes

1 tbsp Herb and garlic soft cheese (such as Boursin)
juice of ½ lime
1 tbsp water
½ × 400g can chickpeas, rinsed and drained
salt and freshly ground black pepper

- Gently heat the cream cheese, lime juice and water in a small frying pan. When the cheese starts to melt, tip in the chickpeas and heat for about 3 minutes, until the chickpeas are warmed through.

- Season generously with salt and pepper. Serve over courgette spaghetti.

COOKING WITH COURGETTE SPAGHETTI

This is a fab range of brilliant recipes that make substantial and filling meals. Some are slow cooked but others take less than half an hour. All provide a filling and tasty and lower calorie dinner.

* * *

Courgette Spaghetti with Roasted Veg

Orange and Lemon Chicken

Best Ever Beef Bolognaise

Monkfish and Chorizo

Hearty Chicken and Bacon

Turkey Meatballs with Tomato Sauce

Prawn Cocktail

Courgette and Feta Fritters

Slow-baked Chicken Rolls

Lentil and Mushroom Bolognaise

Caramelised Onion with Mushrooms

Creamy Purple Sprouting Broccoli

Spicy Butternut Sauce

Quick-cooked Italian Beef and Tomato

Toasted Cumin Halloumi with Butternut Squash

Pork with Pears and Courgette Spaghetti

Grilled Lamb with Fresh Parsley and Mint Sauce

Spanish Baked Prawns

Haddock with Pea and Mint

Buttermilk Chicken

Beef Stroganoff

Chicken Poached in White Wine

Mozzarella and Tomato Salad

Sausage 'Souper' Noodles

Honeyed Chicken Spaghetti

Courgette Spaghetti with Roasted Veg

159 calories

Feel free to mix and match with whatever veggies you find at the bottom of your fridge.

Serves 2 • Ready in 25 minutes

1 yellow pepper, deseeded and cut into chunks
1 red onion, peeled and cut into eighths lengthways
250g butternut squash, peeled, deseeded and cut into chunks
4 medium tomatoes, quartered
2 cloves garlic, unpeeled
1 tsp dried mixed herbs
Salt and freshly ground black pepper
2 tsp olive oil

- Preheat the oven to 220C (200C fan).

- Place all the vegetables, garlic and dried herbs in a large bowl. Add plenty of salt and pepper. Pour over the oil. Toss thoroughly so that all of the vegetables are covered with oil. Transfer to a roasting dish and roast in the oven for 20 minutes.

- Remove the vegetables from the oven and use a fork to squash the garlic cloves firmly, releasing their garlicky juices. Stir through before serving over courgette spaghetti.

Orange and Lemon Chicken

336 calories

A simple but zesty chicken dish.

Serves 2 • Ready in 15 mins

2 skinless chicken breasts
1 tbsp olive oil
Zest and juice of 1 orange
Zest and juice of 1 lemon
½ tsp dried thyme
20g butter
Salt and freshly ground black pepper

- Cut the chicken breasts in half widthways, making two fat pieces. Make a cut about 2.5cm long into the thickest part of each chicken piece. This flattens the chicken slightly allowing it to cook quicker and makes a simple butterfly shape.

- Heat the oil in a frying pan over a medium/high heat. When hot, add the chicken pieces. Sprinkle over the orange and lemon zest and the thyme and season well with salt and pepper. Cook for 4-5 minutes on each side, until golden and just cooked through.

- Add the orange and lemon juices to the pan and allow to sizzle. Reduce the heat to low and let the sauce bubble for 2 minutes. Transfer the chicken to a warm plate.

- Add the butter to the pan and cook over a high heat for 2–4 minutes, until you have a thick glossy sauce. Pour over the chicken and serve immediately.

-

Best Ever Beef Bolognaise

243 calories

This bolognaise sauce is rich and full of flavour. Freeze in batches for easy dinners for you and your family. Watch out though, this makes 12 portions so you'll need a big pan.

Makes 12 portions • Ready in 2 hours 30 minutes

200g bacon, chopped

1 large onion, chopped

1 carrot, peeled and chopped

1 stick celery, diced

1 pepper, deseeded and diced

1 courgette, chopped

1kg lean (10% fat) minced beef

2 x 400g cans chopped tomatoes

2 bay leaves

1 tsp dried mixed herbs

1 tsp salt

1 tbsp tomato puree

1 tsp garlic puree (or 2 cloves fresh, chopped)

1 tbsp tomato ketchup

1 tsp Worcestershire sauce

2 tsp mushroom ketchup

250g mushrooms, washed and sliced

125ml red wine

- Heat a large lidded saucepan and toss in the chopped bacon. When it starts to sizzle, add the onion and fry for 2 mins. Add the carrot and celery, reduce the heat and continue to cook for a few more minutes. Then stir in the pepper and courgette.

- Turn the heat back up to high, then crumble in the minced beef. Continue to stir the meat until it is browned and broken up.

- Reduce the heat to medium and add the chopped tomatoes, bay leaves, dried herbs and salt. Stir, then add the tomato puree, garlic, tomato ketchup, Worcestershire sauce and mushroom ketchup. Stir again.

- Bring up to a gentle simmer, then add the mushrooms and red wine. Bubble for 5 minutes, then turn the heat to the lowest possible setting, put the lid on (slightly ajar) and cook for 2 hours. Alternatively, cook in the oven (lidded) at 160C (150C fan) for 2 hours.

- Cool completely and freeze or refrigerate in 1, 2 or 4 person sizes. Reheat to serve.

Monkfish and Chorizo

191 calories

This dish is so quick to knock up for a one-person lunch or dinner. The flavours really pack a punch too! This would also work well with other types of white fish.

Serves 1 • Ready in 10 minutes

1 large courgette
70g monkfish, cut into slices
½ tsp smoked paprika
20g chorizo, finely sliced
salt and pepper
1 tbsp (15ml) dry white vermouth (Noilly Prat)

- Spiralize and blot the courgette as normal.

- Place the monkfish on a small plate and sprinkle over the paprika and a little salt and pepper, then toss through.

- Heat a small frying pan on a medium-high heat and add the chorizo. Fry for a minute or two, until the juices are released and the chorizo is just starting to turn brown. Add the monkfish and fry for a further minute or two, stirring frequently until cooked through.

- Turn the heat to low, add the vermouth and cook for two minutes. Transfer the contents of the pan to a warmed plate. Leave a little oil in the pan to fry the courgette.

- Return the pan to the heat and turn the temperature

up to high. Add in the blotted courgette and fry, stirring almost continually, for 2-3 minutes.

- Put the courgette in a serving dish and pour the monkfish and sauce over. Serve immediately.

Hearty Chicken and Bacon

312 calories

This sauce can be frozen before the chicken is added.

Serves 4 • Ready in 2 hours 30 minutes

4 slices streaky bacon, roughly chopped
1 onion, peeled and chopped
1 carrot, peeled and diced
1 parsnip, peeled and diced
4 small leeks, washed and sliced
1 red pepper, de-seeded and chopped
salt and pepper to taste
250g chestnut mushrooms, washed and sliced
200ml dry white wine
500ml chicken stock, fresh or made with one cube
2 bay leaves
2 tsp cornflour, mixed to a smooth paste with a little water
400g chicken breast, diced into approx 1 inch cubes

- Pre-heat the oven to 180C/160C fan.

- Heat a large lidded frying pan or oven-proof casserole on a med-high heat on the hob. When hot add the streaky bacon. Fry for 2-3 minutes until just turning brown. Remove the bacon using a slotted spoon and set aside.

- Add the onion to the pan and immediately reduce the heat. Leave the onion to cook slowly in the bacon fat for about 5 minutes.

- Add the carrot, parsnip, leeks and pepper to the pan. Stir thoroughly and season with salt and pepper. Turn the heat up a little and continue to cook for a further 3 minutes.

- Stir through the mushrooms and add the wine and chicken stock. Add the bay leaves and put the bacon back in. Bring to a gentle simmer. Add the cornflour paste and stir continuously until thickened.

- Transfer to an oven-proof dish if necessary.

- Place the lidded dish in the pre-heated oven and cook for approximately 2 hours. You could also cook this dish in a slow cooker for 6-8 hours.

- When you are ready to eat, heat the dish on the hob and bring up to a gentle simmer. If necessary, add a little extra water at this stage. Add the diced chicken and bring back to simmering point. Then cook gently for 12 minutes. Check the chicken is cooked through before serving over courgette spaghetti.

Turkey Meatballs with Tomato Sauce

285 calories

Everyone loves meatballs in tomato sauce. By making the meatballs with turkey mince you are cutting the fat and calories considerably, without any loss of flavour.

Serves 2 • Ready in 45 minutes

1 tsp olive oil

1 garlic clove, peeled and crushed

1 × 400g can chopped tomatoes

1 bay leaf

few leaves of fresh basil, chopped

1 tsp red wine vinegar

250g lean turkey breast mince

1 tsp cornflour

10g (2 tbsp) Parmesan cheese, finely grated

½ tsp dried mixed herbs

few drops Worcestershire sauce

salt and freshly ground black pepper

- In a large, non-stick saucepan heat the oil gently. Stir in the garlic and fry for 1 minute before adding the chopped tomatoes, bay leaf, basil and vinegar. Bring to the boil, reduce the heat and simmer uncovered for 10 minutes.

- Meanwhile, make the meatballs. Put the turkey mince in a large bowl. Add the cornflour, parmesan, mixed herbs, Worcestershire sauce and salt and pepper.

Using your hands, mix all the ingredients well, then form small meatballs. You should get 8–10 balls.

- Drop the meatballs into the sauce and spoon the sauce over them so they are covered. Cook for 20 minutes.

Prawn Cocktail

179 calories

The sweet and reminiscent prawn cocktail makes a delicious sauce for courgette spaghetti.

Serves 1 • Ready in 5 mins

125g cooked king prawns
Juice half a lemon
1 tsp tomato ketchup
1 heaped tsp mayonnaise

- Cook courgette spaghetti as normal. When just cooked, add the king prawns to the pan. Stir and heat through for a minute.
- Combine the lemon juice, ketchup and mayonnaise in a small bowl. Add to the pan and cook through until warmed.

Courgette and Feta Fritters

308 calories

These are so delightful and really easy.

Serves 2 • Ready in 15 minutes

2 large courgettes
3 spring onions, trimmed and finely chopped
100g feta cheese, crumbled
little fresh parsley, chopped (optional)
½ tsp dried mint
½ tsp paprika
salt and freshly ground black pepper
1 level tbsp plain flour
1 large egg, beaten
1 tbsp olive oil

- Spiralize or julienne the courgette as normal and lay out on kitchen paper to dry out. Place another layer of kitchen paper on the top and leave for a few minutes to absorb excess moisture.

- Mix the spring onions, crumbled feta, parsley, mint and paprika in a bowl. Season with salt and pepper and stir in the flour. Pour in the beaten egg and mix well. Finally, mix in the courgette.

- Heat the oil in a wide frying pan over a medium-high heat. When hot, add 1 tablespoon scoops of the mixture to the pan, flattening each scoop with the back of the spoon as you go. The fritters need to be widely spaced so you may have to do this in 2 batches. Fry for about 2 minutes on each side until golden.

Slow-baked Chicken Rolls

396 calories

These stuffed chicken rolls in tomato sauce are great for when you want a substantial dinner. They also freeze well.

Serves 4 • Ready in 2 hours 15 minutes

100g sausagemeat

4 skinless, boneless chicken thighs, about 360g

1 onion, peeled and chopped

2 garlic cloves, peeled and finely chopped

1 red pepper, deseeded and roughly chopped

1 green pepper, deseeded and roughly chopped

1 × 400g can butterbeans, rinsed and drained

1 × 400g can chopped tomatoes

½ chicken stock cube

1 tsp dried oregano

500ml water

- Preheat the oven to 160C/140C fan.
- Divide the sausagemeat into 4 equal portions. Open up the chicken thighs and lay them flat. Place the portion of sausagemeat in the middle of the chicken and pull up the sides so that the meat is enclosed in a tight roll. Attach the two sides of the chicken together with a cocktail stick. Turn the chicken roll over so that the join is on the bottom.

- Use a large casserole dish or slow cooker dish. Layer the onion, garlic and peppers at the base of the dish, then add the butter beans. Place the stuffed chicken thighs on top and pour on the chopped tomatoes. Crunch up the stock cube in your fingers and sprinkle over the top. Add the oregano. Finally, top up with 500ml water or until the chicken is generously covered.
- Cook in the oven for 2 hours. Alternatively, cook in the slow cooker for at least 6 hours.
- Place 4 portions of cooked courgette spaghetti in a large serving dish, add the chicken rolls and pour the sauce over.

Lentil and Mushroom Bolognaise

136 calories

This bolognaise is so filling and versatile that you simply don't need the meat. There is enough here to serve 6 but it freezes well so you can freeze individual portions. Simply re-heat in the microwave for a delicious meal in seconds.

IMPORTANT! Check the packet for the dried lentils before cooking. Some need pre-soaking overnight in cold water. Brown and green lentils generally don't need pre-soaking but it is ALWAYS worth checking.

Serves 6 • Ready in 1 hour

1 tbsp olive oil

1 large onion, chopped

250g mushrooms, washed and sliced

4 cloves garlic, sliced

1 carrot, peeled and chopped

1 green pepper, seeded and chopped

250g brown or green lentils

500ml water

1 bay leaf

2 tbsp tomato puree

1 tbsp (15g) reduced sugar & salt ketchup

1 tsp marmite

1 tsp mushroom ketchup

1 tbsp red wine vinegar

½ tsp chilli flakes

1×400g tin chopped tomatoes

200ml red wine

- In a large pan, heat the oil over a medium heat. Fry the onion for 5 minutes. Add the mushrooms, garlic, carrot and green pepper. Put the lid on the pan and cook for 10 minutes until soft, stirring frequently.

- Stir in the lentils, then add the water, bay leaf, tomato puree, ketchup, marmite, mushroom ketchup, red wine vinegar and chilli flakes. Bring to the boil and cook on a vigorous heat for 10 minutes. Reduce the heat to medium/low, add the chopped tomatoes and wine and cook for a further 20–30 minutes until the sauce is rich and thick.

Caramelised Onion with Mushrooms

268 calories

These sweet and tender onions go beautifully with courgette spaghetti.

Serves 1 • Ready in 30 minutes

1 tsp olive oil
....

1 heaped tsp butter (10g)
....

1 white onion, peeled, halved lengthways and cut into strips
....

½ tsp granulated sugar
....

1 tsp salt
....

150g mushrooms, washed and sliced
....

50g kale, washed and stalks removed
....

Few sprigs fresh rosemary or ½ tsp dried rosemary
....

10g parmesan cheese
....

Freshly ground black pepper
....

- Heat the oil and butter gently in a lidded pan. When the butter has melted, add the onion, sugar and salt. Stir. Turn the heat to the lowest possible setting and cook with the lid on for 15 minutes.

- Remove the lid and turn the heat up to medium. Add the mushroom and cook for 7 minutes before adding the kale for a further 3 minutes. Stir through the parmesan and black pepper just before serving.

Creamy Purple Sprouting Broccoli

171 calories

This delicious sauce for courgette spaghetti is fabulous when purple sprouting broccoli is in season. Also works well with tenderstem broccoli.

Serves 1 • Ready in 15 minutes

1 tsp olive oil
1 shallot, peeled and finely chopped
1 garlic clove, peeled and finely chopped
1 tbsp capers, drained
1 medium tomato, finely chopped
100ml vegetable stock (fresh or made with ¼ cube)
1 tbsp double cream
salt
100g purple sprouting (or tenderstem) broccoli, trimmed

- Heat the oil in a frying pan, add the shallot and gently fry until softened. Add the garlic and cook for 1 min.

- Add the capers, tomato and stock. Bring to the boil, then reduce the heat and simmer gently for 10 minutes. Turn off the heat. If preferred, you can blend the sauce until smooth at this stage. Stir in the cream.

- Meanwhile, bring a saucepan of lightly salted water to the boil and plunge in the broccoli. Cook for 4–6 minutes until just tender.

- Place one portion of cooked courgette spaghetti in a bowl, arrange the broccoli on top and pour over the creamy sauce. Serve immediately.

Spicy Butternut Sauce

104 calories

This delicately spiced sauce is rich and satisfying. It is also suitable for freezing.

Serves 4 • Ready in 30 minutes

1 tsp olive oil
1 onion, peeled and diced
1 red chilli, de-seeded and chopped
½ butternut squash (400g), peeled and diced
1 tsp paprika
1 tsp mild chilli powder
½ tsp ground coriander
1 clove garlic, crushed
salt and pepper
500ml water
1 tbsp (15ml) dry white vermouth (Noilly Prat)
1 tbsp dijon mustard
handful fresh coriander, chopped
4 heaped tsp low fat crème fraiche

- Heat the oil in a large saucepan. Toss in the onion and red chilli and fry gently for 5 minutes. Stir in the butternut squash and add all the spices, garlic and a generous seasoning of salt and pepper. Add the water, bring to the boil and simmer for 20 minutes.

- Remove from the heat and add the Noilly prat and Dijon mustard.

- Transfer to a blender and blend until smooth. Return

to the pan and add the coriander. Reheat gently for 2 minutes before serving over courgette spaghetti. Top with a generous dollop of crème fraiche.

Quick-cooked Italian Beef and Tomato

425 calories

A really special dinner for two.

Serves 2 • Ready in 25 minutes

2 tsp olive oil

200g beef rump steak

salt and freshly ground black pepper

½ onion, peeled and sliced into half rings

1 garlic clove, peeled and thinly sliced

½ green pepper, deseeded and sliced

½ yellow pepper, deseeded and sliced

4 medium tomatoes, roughly chopped

1 tbsp tomato puree

100ml water

½ tsp dried mixed herbs

a little fresh oregano

12 large black olives, pitted

- Use a very sharp knife to cut thin slivers of the beef.

- Heat the oil in a large pan over a high heat. Season the beef with salt and pepper. When the oil is hot, toss in the beef and stir-fry for 2 minutes or until seared all over. Remove the beef from the pan and set aside.

- Reduce the heat to medium and fry the onion, garlic and peppers for 5–10 minutes until tender. With the heat still at medium, add the tomatoes, tomato puree, water and herbs and simmer for 10 minutes.

- Stir through the beef strips and olives and heat for a further 2 minutes before serving.

Toasted Cumin Halloumi with Butternut Squash

333 calories

This unusual dish has a North African feel to it, with the touch of heat tempered by the sweetness of the butternut squash and the saltiness of the halloumi.

Serves 2 • Ready in 15 minutes

300g (½ small) butternut squash, peeled and cut into large chunks
1 tsp cumin seeds
1 tsp chilli flakes
1 tbsp olive oil
2 tsp tomato purée
1 tsp garlic purée (or 1 clove, crushed)
120g halloumi, cut into chunks
1 spring onion, trimmed and chopped
50g piquante peppers from a jar, drained and chopped
Juice of 1 lime
Freshly ground black pepper
Handful of fresh coriander, chopped (optional)

- Put the cubed butternut squash into a microwaveable dish, cover and microwave for 5 minutes on high.

- Place a frying pan over a medium/high heat and toss in the cumin seeds and chilli flakes. Dry fry for one minute, then reduce the heat to medium and add the oil, tomato purée and garlic. Stir for a few seconds before adding the halloumi and spring onions. Stir-fry for 3 minutes.

- Add the peppers and butternut squash and continue to cook, stirring regularly, until browned on all sides. Remove from the heat and stir in the lime juice, black pepper and coriander. Serve immediately over courgette spaghetti.

Pork with Pears and Courgette Spaghetti

385 calories

This sweet and salty pork dish is a treat for any occasion.

Serves 2 • Ready in 15 minutes

2 × 100g lean pork steaks
....
salt and freshly ground black pepper
....
20g walnuts, roughly chopped
....
1 tsp olive oil
....
2 shallots, peeled and cut into eighths
....
2 pears, quartered and cored
....
1 tsp runny honey
....
1 fresh rosemary sprig (or ½ tsp dried)
....

- Cover the pork steaks with cling film and bash with a rolling pin until half their original thickness. Season well with salt and pepper.

- Heat a wide frying pan over a high heat. Toss in the walnuts and toast for about 2 minutes, shaking once or twice to make sure they are evenly toasted. Remove to a plate and set aside.

- Add the oil and shallots to the pan and reduce the heat to medium. Fry the shallots for 3 minutes before adding the pears, honey and rosemary. Cook for another 3–5 minutes until starting to caramelise. Remove to a plate and set aside.

- Add the pork steaks to the pan. Fry for 5–8 minutes, turning once until browned and cooked to your liking. Reintroduce the pears and simmer gently for a further minute.

- Arrange the cooked courgette spaghetti over 2 plates. Add the pork steaks and the pear mixtures. Serve with the toasted walnuts sprinkled over.

Grilled Lamb with Fresh Parsley and Mint Sauce

309 calories

You really need some fresh parsley and mint for this sauce but it is definitely worth it. Prepare the sauce first, it works better if the flavours are left to combine for a few minutes. The sauce keeps well in the fridge for a few days.

Serves 2 • Ready in 20 minutes

1 garlic clove, peeled
....
salt and freshly ground black pepper
....
2 fresh mint leaves
....
large bunch of flat-leaf (Italian) parsley
....
juice of 1 lemon
....
2 tbsp extra virgin olive oil
....
2 × 100g lean lamb leg steaks
....

- Place the garlic, salt & pepper, the herbs and lemon juice in a blender and process until they form a paste. If you don't have a blender, you can chop the ingredients finely instead. Gradually pour in the olive oil, blending until it forms a smooth thick sauce. Transfer the sauce to a wide dish that is big enough to hold the lamb.

- Preheat the grill to medium-high. Season the lamb and place under the grill. Cook for 5–8 minutes on each side, depending on how you like your lamb. It should be seared on the outside and if you like it a little pink, you should make sure the inside gets properly hot, that's 145C on a meat thermometer.

- Transfer the lamb to the serving dish and scoop up the sauce over the top. Leave to rest in the sauce for a few minutes before serving over courgette spaghetti.

Spanish Baked Prawns

251 calories

I love this easy prawn dish. You can use fresh or frozen prawns so it really is a no-brainer!

Serves 2 • Ready in 15 minutes

2 tbsp extra-virgin olive oil

2 tbsp tomato purée

1 red chilli, seeded and finely chopped

2 cloves garlic, crushed

1 tsp paprika

½ tsp dried dill or 1 tsp fresh

2 tbsp white wine vinegar

Few drops of Tabasco

200ml passata

250g cooked and peeled prawns (fresh or frozen)

- Preheat the oven to 230C/210C fan.
- In a small bowl or jug mix together the olive oil, tomato purée, chilli, garlic, paprika, dill, white wine vinegar, Tabasco and passata.
- Arrange the prawns in a small baking dish and pour the dressing over. Bake in the oven for 7 minutes for fresh prawns or 10 minutes for frozen.

Haddock with Pea and Mint

317 calories

Serves 2 • Ready in 20 minutes

2 x 150g skinless and boneless haddock pieces
....
2 tsp olive oil
....
salt and freshly ground black pepper
....
2 spring onions, trimmed and roughly chopped
....
½ iceberg lettuce, outer leaves removed and roughly chopped
....
200g frozen peas
....
400ml fresh vegetable or fish stock
....
4 fresh mint leaves
....
50g Greek yogurt
....
freshly ground black pepper
....

- Preheat the oven to 200C/180C fan.

- Place the fish on a baking tray, season well with salt and pepper and rub over 1 tsp of the olive oil. Bake for 15-20 minutes until cooked and slightly flaky.

- In a large saucepan, heat the oil over a low heat. Stir in the spring onions and lettuce for 1–2 minutes until the lettuce starts to wilt. Add the peas, stock and mint leaves. Bring to a gentle simmer and cook for 10 minutes or until all the vegetables are tender. Blend until smooth. For an even smoother texture, pass the soup through a sieve after blending.

- Return to the sauce to the pan, stir in the yogurt and bring back up to temperature. Add a little more salt and pepper if necessary.

- Place cooked courgette spaghetti in a serving dish, add the fish and pour over the sauce.

Buttermilk Chicken

212 calories

Marinating the chicken in buttermilk for just half an hour gives the chicken a delicious succulence.

Serves 2 • Ready in 45 minutes

150ml buttermilk
....
2 garlic cloves, peeled and crushed
....
salt and freshly ground black pepper
....
2 × 150g skinless chicken breasts, halved
....
1 tsp olive oil
....

- Place the buttermilk in a wide bowl and stir in the garlic and salt and pepper.

- Lightly score the chicken breasts, then submerge in the buttermilk. Turn the chicken in the sauce to make sure it is fully covered. Cover the bowl with clingfilm, then chill for 30 minutes or more.

- When you are ready to cook the chicken, heat the oil in a frying pan on a med-high heat. Remove the chicken from the marinade and place in the frying pan. Fry the chicken for 5-6 minutes each side until cooked through. Remove the chicken from the pan and place the chicken on your cooked courgette spaghetti. Add the remaining marinade to the pan and bubble for 2 minutes before pouring over the chicken.

Beef Stroganoff

428 calories

This is a fab recipe and goes exceptionally well with courgette spaghetti. Try cutting the courgette into fat ribbons using a vegetable peeler to make pappardelle pasta.

Serves 2 • Ready in 15 minutes

200g trimmed fillet or rump steak
1 tbsp olive oil
10g butter
1 shallot, peeled and sliced
1 clove garlic, finely chopped
200g mushrooms, washed and sliced
1 tbsp cooking sherry
1 tsp paprika
1 tsp Dijon mustard
1 tsp tomato puree
1 tsp cornflour
100ml water
2 tbsp crème fraiche
Salt and freshly ground black pepper

- Using a very sharp knife, cut very thin slices of the beef steak. Heat the oil in a wide frying pan on a high heat. Toss in the steak slices and quickly sear the beef until browned on both sides. Remove the meat from the pan and set aside to rest.

- Turn the heat down to medium, then add the butter. When the butter has melted, add the shallot, garlic and mushrooms. Stir-fry for a few minutes until the mushrooms are soft and glossy.

- Reduce the heat to low and splash in the sherry. Stir in the paprika, Dijon mustard, tomato puree and cornflour. Slowly add the water, stirring continuously, until the sauce starts to thicken. Bring to a really gentle simmer and cook for 5 minutes. Add the crème fraiche and put the beef back in. Warm through for 2 minutes before serving.

Chicken Poached in White Wine

264 calories

A lovely easy dinner for one.

Serves 1 • Ready in 15 minutes

1 tsp olive oil
....
½ garlic clove, peeled and crushed
....
2 spring onions, trimmed and sliced
....
½ tsp dried mixed herbs
....
1 × 150g skinless chicken breast, halved
....
100ml dry white wine
....
1 tbsp light soft cheese
....
small handful of fresh parsley, chopped
....

- Heat the oil, garlic, spring onions and dried mixed herbs in a small lidded frying pan or saucepan for 1–2 minutes until sizzling. Add the chicken and cook for about 5 minutes until the first side turns golden.

- Turn the chicken over and add the white wine. Put the lid on and turn the heat to low. Let the chicken continue to cook in the wine for a further 5-8 minutes. Check that the chicken is cooked through before removing from the pan and covering.

- Bring the remaining liquid in the pan back up to simmering and stir in the soft cheese. Bubble for 2–3 minutes until you get a pleasingly thick sauce. Stir in the parsley and pour over the chicken.

Mozzarella and Tomato Salad

342 calories

In this recipe you lightly cook the courgette and mix with a dressing to make a salad.

Serves 1 • Ready in 7 minutes

1 tsp olive oil

½ clove garlic, peeled and crushed

1 large or 2 small courgettes, spiralized or julienned

10 cherry tomatoes, quartered

zest and juice of ½ lemon

1 tbsp balsamic vinegar

1 tsp extra virgin olive oil

salt and freshly ground black pepper

5 fresh basil leaves

½ ball Italian mozzarella (75g)

- In a wide frying pan, heat the olive oil over a medium–high heat. When hot, toss in the garlic and fry for 1 minute. Add the courgette, then season with salt and pepper and cook for 2 minutes. Give it a stir and cook for a further 1–2 minutes or until the courgette is cooked through yet firm.

- Mix the tomatoes, lemon zest, lemon juice, balsamic vinegar and extra virgin olive oil together in a large bowl. Add the cooked courgette and stir through. Leave to stand for a few minutes.

- Transfer the courgette to a serving bowl bowl or plate. Tear the basil and mozzarella and arrange over the top. Serve immediately.

Sausage 'Souper' Noodles

295 calories

A warming and reassuring noodle soup for a rainy evening.

Serves 2 • Ready in 45 minutes

1 litre fresh chicken stock

1 leek, trimmed and sliced

2 large Cumberland sausages, sliced into 2cm pieces

1 red chilli, deseeded and sliced

1 parmesan rind (for flavour only, removed after cooking)

2 bay leaves

½ tsp dried mixed herbs or small handful of fresh basil and/or parsley if available

100g soya (edamame) beans, fresh or frozen

2 medium tomatoes, diced

salt and freshly ground black pepper

10g (2 tsp) fresh parmesan, grated

- Heat the chicken stock in a large saucepan with the leek, sausages, chilli, Parmesan rind, bay leaves and dried herbs. Bring to a gentle simmer and cook for about 25 minutes.

- Add the soya beans and simmer for a further 10 minutes.

- Remove the Parmesan rind and bay leaves from the pan and add the tomatoes and any fresh herbs if using.

- Serve over courgette spaghetti in large bowls and season generously. Sprinkle the grated Parmesan over the top.

Honeyed Chicken Spaghetti

334 calories

Serves 1 • Ready in 15 minutes

1 tsp olive oil

1 large courgette, julienned or spiralized

juice of ½ lemon

1 tsp balsamic vinegar

1 tsp extra virgin olive oil

1 tsp runny honey

salt and freshly ground black pepper

1 tsp (5g) butter

1 × 150g skinless chicken breast, diced

80g broccoli, cut into small florets

- Begin by preparing your serving dish. It should be wide with a lip and able to hold the chicken, courgette spaghetti and broccoli comfortably. Put the lemon juice, vinegar, extra virgin olive oil, honey and salt and pepper in the dish and whisk together with a fork. Set aside.

- Prepare the courgette spaghetti as normal but only lightly cook. Stir into the lemon juice and vinegar.

- Re-use the frying pan from the courgette, adding the butter. When the butter has melted, add the chicken pieces and fry for 10-12 minutes, turning once, until golden and cooked through. As soon as it is cooked, transfer to the serving dish and toss into the dressing.

- Meanwhile, bring a pan of water to the boil and plunge in the broccoli. Cook for 6 minutes until tender. Drain and combine with the courgette spaghetti, chicken and dressing.

- Leave the dish for 2 minutes before serving to allow the flavours to combine.

THE NOODLE BAR

First of all, let's be clear. Courgette noodles are exactly the same base ingredient as courgette spaghetti AND you prepare them in an identical way. The difference is just in their usage. Courgette spaghetti for all things Italian, European or with a similar pasta equivalent. Courgette noodles (or zoodles as the Americans call them) are used in Asian and Chinese dishes and anything remotely Eastern.

• • •

Chinese-style Pork Noodles

Japanese Beef & Prawn Noodles

Caribbean Chicken Noodles

Chowder noodles

Spicy Lamb Keema Noodles

Thai baked salmon

Pad Thai

Spicy Pork Chilli Noodles

Sweet Tomato Soup Noodles

Chinese Chicken Stir-fry

Thai Coconut Noodles

Yellow Noodles with Cauliflower

Crab Cakes with Coconut Noodles

Harissa Chickpea Noodles

Indian Green Soup Noodles

Chinese-style Pork Noodles

387 calories

There is so much flavour in these delicious noodles.

Serves 2 • Ready in 20 minutes

200g firm tofu, cut into large cubes

1 tsp cornflour

2 tbsp water

1 tbsp rice wine

1 tbsp tomato purée

1 tsp brown sugar

1 tbsp soy sauce

1 clove garlic, peeled and crushed

1 thumb (5cm) fresh ginger, peeled and grated

2 tsp olive oil

50g shiitake mushrooms, sliced

1 shallot, peeled and sliced

2 large courgettes, julienned or spiralized

200g pork mince (10% fat)

50g beansprouts

- Lay out the tofu on kitchen paper, cover with more kitchen paper and set aside.
- In a small bowl, mix together the cornflour and water, removing all lumps, rice wine, tomato purée, brown sugar and soy sauce. Add the crushed garlic and ginger and stir together.
- In a wok or large frying pan, heat the oil to a high temperature. Add the shiitake mushrooms and stir-fry

for 2–3 minutes until cooked and glossy. Remove the mushrooms from the pan with a slotted spoon and set aside. Add the tofu to the pan and stir-fry until golden on all sides. Remove with a slotted spoon and set aside.

- Add the shallot and spiralized courgette to the wok, stir-fry for 2 minutes, then add the mince. cook until the mince is cooked through, then add the sauce, reduce the heat a notch and allow the sauce to bubble round the meat for a minute or two. Add the beansprouts, shiitake mushrooms and tofu to the pan and warm through. Remove from the heat and serve immediately.

Japanese Beef & Prawn Noodles

257 calories

This is an amazingly tasty dish. So full of flavour, the whole family will love it.

Serves 4 • Ready in 20 minutes

1 tbsp olive oil
5 medium courgettes, julienned or spiralized
200g minced beef
2 tsp Chinese five-spice powder
2 cloves garlic, finely grated
1 large thumb-sized piece of ginger, peeled and finely grated
250g cooked king prawns
2 heaped tsp brown sugar
6 spring onions, trimmed and finely sliced
Juice of 1 lime
1 tsp nam pla fish sauce
2 tsp soy sauce
1 red chilli, deseeded and finely sliced
Handful of fresh coriander, chopped
2 fresh mint leaves, chopped
Freshly ground black pepper

- In a wok or large frying pan, fry the spiralized courgette as normal to make courgette spaghetti. Remove the cooked courgette from the pan and set aside.
- Heat the same pan over a medium heat and add the

minced beef and five-spice powder. Fry until well browned. Add the garlic, ginger, prawns, brown sugar and spring onions. Cook for 3–4 minutes.

- Place the courgette noodles in a large bowl with the lime juice, nam pla, soy sauce, red chilli, coriander, mint and black pepper. Stir through and divide between four plates. Serve the beef and prawn mixture over the noodles.

Caribbean Chicken Noodles

256 calories

This thick Caribbean sauce is highly addictive.

Serves 2 • Ready in 15 minutes

1 tsp dark brown sugar
¼ tsp smoked paprika
½ tsp dried oregano
1 tsp cornflour
1 tsp Dijon mustard
½ tsp maple syrup
¼ tsp Worcestershire sauce
1 tsp cider vinegar
½ tsp black treacle
pinch of salt
2 × 150g skinless chicken breasts, halved and scored lightly with a knife
2 tsp olive oil
2 large courgettes, julienned or spiralized

- Preheat the grill to a medium–high setting.

- Simply mix together the sugar, paprika, oregano, mustard, maple syrup, Worcestershire sauce, cider vinegar, black treacle and a pinch of salt in a small bowl. Add a little water if necessary to make it into a spreadable consistency.

- Spread the mixture over the chicken breasts, making sure you coat all sides. Retain any remaining sauce to add to the noodles.

- Grill the chicken for 5–7 minutes on each side

depending on thickness and check that the chicken is cooked through before serving.

- Fry the courgette in the olive oil and when cooked add any remaining marinade and allow to bubble around the courgette for 2-3 minutes. Serve with the grilled chicken arranged over the top.

Chowder noodles

370 calories

This is low-calorie comfort food and is perfect for warming you up on a wet day.

Serves 1 • Ready in 25 minutes

2 black peppercorns

1 bay leaf

100g skinless smoked haddock or cod

150ml milk

250ml fish or vegetable stock (fresh or made with ½ cube)

1 tsp olive oil

1 large or 2 medium courgettes, julienned or spiralized

1 small carrot, julienned or spiralized

1 leek, trimmed and cut into thin rings

½ tsp cumin seeds

1 tbsp double cream

• Place the peppercorns, bay leaf and fish in a saucepan. Pour in the milk and stock and bring to a gentle simmer. Continue to simmer gently until just cooked through, about 6–8 minutes. Remove the fish from the pan and set aside, reserving the cooking liquid.

• Meanwhile in a wide lidded frying pan, heat the oil on a med-high setting and cook the courgette and carrot noodles as normal. Remove to kitchen paper. Turn the heat to low and stir in the leeks. Put the lid on and soften the leeks for 10 minutes.

• Remove the lid from the leeks and turn up the heat.

Add the cumin seeds and fry until they start to sizzle and pop. Pour in the poaching liquid from the fish and bring to the boil. Simmer for 5 minutes.

- Turn off the heat and stir in the courgette and carrot noodles. Break the fish apart gently with your fingers and add to the pan. Stir in the cream and heat gently for 1–2 minutes before serving.

Spicy Lamb Keema Noodles

457 calories

This is quick and easy to rustle up after work.

Serves 2 • Ready in 30 minutes

2 tbsp mirin

1 tsp honey

1 tsp miso paste

1 tsp mild chilli powder

1 tbsp dark soy sauce

200g lean minced lamb

1 tsp olive oil

4 spring onions, chopped

2 large courgettes, julienned or spiralized

1 carrot, julienned or spiralized

100g peas, fresh or frozen

handful of fresh coriander (optional), chopped

- Mix together the mirin, honey, miso paste, chilli powder and soy sauce.

- Break the lamb apart with your fingers and put into a large bowl. Pour the sauce over and mix together. Leave to marinate for 5–10 minutes.

- Meanwhile, heat the oil in a large frying pan over a medium-high heat. When hot, toss in the spring onions, courgette and carrot and stir-fry until just tender.

- Tip any extra sauce out of the lamb and set aside for later. Add the lamb to the pan and stir-fry until brown all over. Stir in the peas.

- Add 100ml water, bring up to a simmer then reduce the heat to low. Add any remaining sauce from the meat and cook for 15 minutes. Add the carrot and courgette noodles back to the pan.
- Stir in the chopped coriander before serving.

Thai baked salmon

309 calories

Using pre-made lemongrass and ginger pastes
simplifies the making of this dish.

Serves 2 • Ready in 20 minutes

handful of fresh coriander, chopped

zest and juice of ½ lime

½ lemongrass stalk, shredded or 1 tsp
lemongrass purée

1 cm piece of fresh ginger, peeled and
grated or 1 tsp ginger purée

½ tsp mild chilli powder

1 tsp palm sugar or brown sugar

pinch of salt

2 skinless salmon fillets, about 130g each

2 tsp olive oil

2 large courgettes, julienned or spiralized

juice of half a lime

- Preheat the oven to 200C/180C fan.

- Mix the coriander, lime zest and juice, lemongrass,
  ginger, chilli powder, sugar and a little salt together
  in a small bowl.

- Place the salmon fillets on a baking tray and rub the
  herb and spice mixture all over the top and sides of
  the salmon.

- Bake in the oven for 18–20 minutes until the salmon
  is just cooked through.

- Five minutes before the salmon is ready, heat the
  oil in a wide frying pan and stir-fry the courgette to

make a batch of courgette noodles. Stir through the lime juice just after cooking. Serve the salmon on top of a bed of fresh courgette noodles.

Pad Thai

406 calories

The courgette noodles make a great substitute for traditional rice noodles.

Serves 2 • Ready in 20 minutes

1 tsp brown sugar
....
Juice of 1 lime
....
200g chicken breast, thinly sliced
....
1 tbsp rice wine vinegar
....
1 tbsp water
....
1 tbsp soy sauce
....
1 tbsp nam pla (fish sauce)
....
2 large eggs
....
Pinch of salt
....
2 tbsp olive oil
....
1 chilli, seeded and diced
....
1 clove garlic, finely chopped
....
1 small thumb-sized piece of ginger, peeled and cut into thin matchsticks
....
3 spring onions, trimmed and sliced
....
2 large courgettes, spiralized or julienned and dried on kitchen towels
....
½ carrot, peeled and spiralized
....
100g beansprouts
....
Handful of fresh coriander, chopped
....
Extra lime wedges, to serve
....

• Place the brown sugar and lime juice in a bowl and toss in the sliced chicken. Mix it all together and set aside to rest.

- In a small dish mix together the rice wine vinegar, water, soy sauce and nam pla. In a separate bowl, whisk the eggs lightly with the salt.

- Heat the oil in a wok or large frying pan over a high heat. Add the chilli, garlic, ginger and half the spring onions and fry for 1 minute before tossing in the chicken, together with its marinade. Stir-fry until the chicken is nearly cooked. Pour in the beaten eggs and let it cook until the egg mixture sets around the chicken and the chicken is cooked through. Then break up the egg by stirring thoroughly; transfer the eggs and chicken to a plate.

- Return the wok to the heat and toss in the spiralized courgette and carrot. Add the beansprouts and remaining spring onions. Stir-fry for several minutes until cooked. Add the soy sauce mixture and stir through for a minute or two before adding the chicken and egg mixture. Stir for another minute before adding the coriander. Serve immediately with a wedge of lime on the side.

Spicy Pork Chilli Noodles

391 calories

A warming and filling winter dish.

Serves 2 • Ready in 25 minutes

1 tsp olive oil

1 shallot, chopped

½ green pepper, deseeded and chopped

1 tsp caraway seeds

1 clove garlic, thinly sliced

300g lean pork mince (10% fat)

½ tsp nutmeg

1 heaped tsp paprika

1 tsp smoked paprika

1 tbsp tomato puree

2 medium tomatoes, chopped

2 tbsp water

Salt and freshly ground black pepper

1 tsp olive oil

2 large courgettes, julienned or spiralized

- Heat the oil in a large pan or casserole dish. Toss in the shallot, green pepper and caraway seeds. Fry lightly for 5 minutes before adding the garlic. Cook for a further 2 minutes.

- Break up the mince with your hands and drop it into the pan. Sprinkle over the rest of the spices and tomato puree and season generously with salt and pepper. Turn the heat up and stir continuously until the meat is cooked through.

- Reduce the heat and add the tomatoes and water. Cook slowly for 10 minutes. Remove the cooked pork from the pan.
- Add another tsp of olive oil to the pan and cook the courgette noodles as normal. When cooked, stir in the smoked pork chilli. Serve immediately.

Sweet Tomato Soup Noodles

148 calories

Sweet and savoury. You can also add prawns to this dish to make a bigger meal.

Serves 1 • Ready in 10 minutes

1 tsp olive oil

½ stick cinnamon

½ tsp cumin seeds

1 bay leaf

1 clove

1 shallot, finely chopped

½ red pepper, deseeded and finely chopped

1 red chilli, deseeded and chopped

1 large or 2 small courgettes, julienned or spiralized

2 cloves garlic, very finely sliced

½ tsp mild chilli powder

½ tsp paprika

¼ tsp ground coriander

½ tsp salt

2 tomatoes, chopped

400ml water

Freshly ground black pepper

• Heat the oil in a heavy-based wide pan. Add the cinnamon, cumin seeds, bay leaf and cloves. Fry for 1 minute, or until they just start to release their aroma. Add the onion, red pepper and chilli and cook on a low heat for 5 minutes. Turn the heat up to high, add the courgette and stir-fry 2-3 minutes.

- Add the garlic, chilli powder, paprika, coriander, salt and tomatoes. Add the water and bring up to a simmer. Cook for a further 5 minutes. Check the seasoning and add more salt and pepper if necessary.

- Remove the cinnamon stick, bay leaf and cloves and serve in a deep bowl.

Chinese Chicken Stir-fry

389 calories

Coating the chicken in cornflour is a traditional Chinese technique which gives the chicken a great succulent flavour.

Serves 1 • Ready in 15 minutes

1 small skinless chicken breast (125g), cut into strips
....

1 tsp cornflour
....

1 tsp water
....

1 tsp rice wine
....

1 tsp tomato puree
....

½ tsp brown sugar
....

1 tbsp light soy sauce
....

½ clove garlic, peeled and grated
....

½ thumb (2cm) fresh ginger, peeled and grated
....

1 tsp olive oil
....

½ tsp walnut oil
....

50g shiitake mushrooms, sliced
....

2 spring onions, trimmed and shredded
....

100g pak choi, stalks spiralized
....

1 small carrot, peeled and spiralized
....

1 small courgette,trimmed and spiralized
....

• Toss the chicken pieces in the cornflour until they are fully coated. Set aside. In a small bowl, stir together the water, rice wine, tomato puree, brown sugar and soy sauce. Add the garlic and ginger and stir together.

- In a wok or large frying pan, heat the olive and walnut oils together on a medium heat. Add the chicken and stir-fry for 4-5 minutes each side until cooked through. Remove the chicken from the pan with a slotted spoon and set aside.

- Turn the heat up to high, add the shiitake mushrooms to the pan and stir-fry for 2-3 minutes until cooked and glossy. Then add the spring onions, pak choi (leaves and spiralized stalks), carrot and courgette and stir-fry until the pak choi leaves have wilted.

- Reduce the heat to low, then stir in the cooked chicken. Add the sauce and allow the sauce to bubble around the chicken for a minute. Remove from the heat and serve immediately.

Thai Coconut Noodles

382 calories

Good comfort food.

Serves 1 • Ready in 15 minutes

1 tsp olive oil

100g pak choi, trimmed and washed, stalks spiralized

1 large or 2 small courgettes, julienned or spiralized

100g shiitake mushrooms, washed and sliced

1 tsp walnut oil

1 tsp fish sauce

Zest of 1 lime

¼ x 400-g tin coconut milk

200ml water

Juice of ½ lime

- Cut the leaves off the pak choi and save for later. Spiralize the pak choi stems. Heat the olive oil in a wide, deep frying pan. Add the spiralized pak choi and courgette. Stir-fry over a high heat until tender, about 3 minutes. Remove the pak choi and courgette from the pan and set aside. Add the mushrooms and stir-fry for 3 minutes until glossy. Stir through the walnut oil, fish sauce and the lime zest.

- Roughly chop the pak choi leaves and add to the pan. From the tin of coconut milk, add about 2 tablespoons of the thick creamy bit from the top and two tablespoon of the coconut water from the bottom. Add the water. Stir in and cook until bubbling.

Simmer for 5 minutes.

- Remove from the heat and add the courgette and lime juice. Serve immediately in a wide bowl.

Yellow Noodles with Cauliflower

144 calories

These noodles are simply full of good flavours.

Serves 1 • Ready in 15 minutes

¼ tsp cumin seeds

¼ tsp coriander seeds

1 cardamom pod

1 tsp olive oil

1 shallot, finely chopped

½ yellow pepper, deseeded and chopped

100g cauliflower, cut into small florets

¼ tsp turmeric

2 strands saffron

1 large courgette, julienned or spiralized

Salt and freshly ground black pepper

- Crush the cumin seeds, coriander seeds and cardamom pod in a pestle and mortar. Heat a heavy-based frying pan over a high heat and dry fry these spices for 1 minute.

- Turn the heat right down and add the oil, shallot, yellow pepper and cauliflower. Fry slowly until soft and translucent, about 10 minutes. Add the rest of the spices, salt and pepper and stir through. Turn the heat to high and add the noodles. Stir-fry until tender.

Crab Cakes with Coconut Noodles

376 calories

Perfect for guests or just when you fancy treating yourself.

Serves 1 • Ready in 15 minutes

1 × 170g can white crabmeat, drained (120g drained weight)

....

1 tbsp plain flour

....

1 tbsp desiccated coconut

....

2 slices jalapeño peppers (from a jar), chopped

....

pinch of sugar

....

juice of ½ lime

....

1 tsp olive oil

....

For the noodles:

....

1 tbsp desiccated coconut

....

1 large courgette, julienned or spiralized

....

1 tsp fish sauce

....

1 tbsp coconut cream

....

juice of half a lime

....

- Combine the crabmeat, flour, coconut, jalapeños, sugar and lime juice in a bowl, then form the mixture into 4–6 small balls. Place the balls on a baking tray and press down gently with the back of a fork to make a small patty. If you have time, cover with clingfilm and chill about 30 minutes.

- Heat the oil in a wide non-stick frying pan over a high heat. When hot, lift the patties into the pan, leaving as much space as you can between them, and cook for

1-2 minute on each side. They should be pleasingly golden and heated right through inside. Remove from the pan and set aside.

- Add the desiccated coconut to the pan, fry for just a minute until just starting to be tinged golden, then add the courgette noodles. Stir fry until cooked and tender. Stir in the fish sauce, coconut cream and lime juice until well combined and lightly bubbling.

Harissa Chickpea Noodles

266 calories

Chickpeas are a good source of protein and surprisingly nutty and filling. Here's a great way to make a sparkling vegetarian dish.

Serves 1 • Ready in 8 minutes

| 1 tsp olive oil |
| 1 large courgette, julienned or spiralized |
| 1 carrot, julienned or spiralized |
| 1 heaped tsp harissa paste |
| 1 heaped tsp tomato purée |
| ½ × 400g can chickpeas, rinsed and drained |
| juice of ½ lemon |

- Heat the olive oil in a frying pan on a high setting and add the spiralized courgette & carrot. Cook for 2m.
- Add the harissa and tomato purée and cook for a further minute or two, until sizzling. Reduce the heat to low and stir in the chickpeas and lemon juice. Cook for 2–3 minutes, until warmed through.

Indian Green Soup Noodles

169 calories

This light meal has got a bit of a heat hit to warm you up.

Serves 1 • Ready in 10 minutes

50g spinach, fresh or frozen

50g peas, fresh or frozen

1 tsp olive oil

1 shallot, chopped

1 bird's eye chilli, finely chopped

1 large or 2 small courgettes, julienned or spiralized

½ tsp aniseed seeds

500ml chicken or vegetable stock

½ tsp garam masala

½ tsp ground cumin

Salt and freshly ground black pepper

- Place the spinach and peas in a microwave-safe bowl and cover with cling film, leaving a 2cm gap at the side for steam to escape. Cook for about 3 minutes if using fresh or 5 minutes from frozen. Set aside to cool.

- Heat the oil in a heavy-based wide pan over a med-high heat. Add the shallot, chilli, courgettes and aniseed seeds. Cook 2 minutes then add the stock. Bring to a simmer and cook for 5 minutes.

- Add the garam masala & cumin and stir through. Add the spinach and peas and cook until warmed through. Season with salt & pepper and serve in a large bowl.

CUCUMBER NOODLES

Cucumber noodles make fantastic and easy salads. Cucumber can be peeled first or spiralized skin on.

As the noodles can be watery, the flavour and texture are both improved by blotting on kitchen paper, using a similar sandwich technique to the courgette spaghetti, for a few minutes before serving.

• • •

Goat's Cheese Salad

Strawberry and Avocado Salad

Smoked Salmon with Soft-boiled Egg

Sesame Chicken Noodles

Cucumber and Asparagus Salad with Prosciutto

Superfood Salad Bowl

Cucumber Egg Florentine

Oriental Salmon Fishcakes on Lime Noodles

Japanese-style Sake Prawn Salad

Tinned Salmon and Bean Salad

Paprika Chicken Noodles

Avocado and Bacon Salad

Lime Salsa Prawns

Creamy Cucumber Noodles with Baked Salmon

Smoked Mackerel and Lentils

Garlic Butter Chicken

Pomegranate, Feta and Walnut Salad

Goat's Cheese Salad

383 calories

This salty and sweet salad is hard to beat on a sunny day.

Serves 2 • Ready in 5 minutes

40g pine nuts

1 cucumber, spiralized and blotted on kitchen paper

100g goat's cheese

40g young spinach leaves

A few fresh basil leaves, torn

1 tbsp extra virgin olive oil

1 tbsp balsamic vinegar

Salt and freshly ground black pepper

- Place the pine nuts in a frying pan and heat on a high heat for about 2 minutes, tipping the pan from side to side frequently to avoid burning. When lightly toasted tip onto a small plate to cool.

- Gently toss the cucumber noodles with the goat's cheese, spinach leaves and basil. Arrange the salad over 2 plates.

- In a small bowl, mix the olive oil, balsamic vinegar and salt and pepper together. Pour over the salad plates and finally add the toasted pine nuts.

Strawberry and Avocado Salad

299 calories

Very summery. The strawberry and feta combination
is divine.

Serves 2 • Ready in 5 minutes

1 cucumber, spiralized and blotted on
kitchen paper

100g strawberries, hulled, washed and
chopped

50g feta cheese

20g walnuts, roughly chopped

½ avocado, peeled, stoned and chopped

1 tbsp extra virgin olive oil

1 tbsp cider vinegar

Pinch of salt and freshly ground black
pepper

- Place the cucumber in a large bowl and gently toss
through the strawberries, feta, walnuts and avocado.

- In a small bowl, mix the olive oil, cider vinegar and
salt and pepper. Pour over the salad, mix gently and
distribute between 2 plates.

Smoked Salmon with Soft-boiled Egg

337 calories

This dish is simple to throw together and is stack full of protein to fill you up. Smoked salmon gives it a luxurious feel.

Makes 1 portion • Ready in 10 minutes

1 large egg
....
2 tsp extra virgin olive oil
....
½ tsp English mustard
....
pinch of sugar
....
1 tsp mayonnaise
....
juice of half lemon
....
salt and pepper
....
½ cucumber, spiralized and blotted on kitchen paper
....
10g baby leaf spinach
....
60g smoked salmon, cut into small thin slices
....

- Heat a small pan of water to boiling. Using a slotted spoon, gently lower the egg into the boiling water. Heat for 8-10 minutes depending on how well-cooked you like your egg. Remove from the water using the slotted spoon and cool in a bowl of cold water for a minute or two to stop the cooking process.

- Meanwhile, make the dressing by combining the olive oil, mustard, sugar, mayonnaise, lemon juice and salt and pepper in a small bowl.

- Arrange the spiralized cucumber and spinach over

a plate and pour over half the dressing. Add the salmon. Peel the just cooled egg and quarter. Arrange the egg pieces over the salmon. Drizzle the rest of the dressing over. Serve immediately.

Sesame Chicken Noodles

303 calories

Fresh, unusual and tasty.

Serves 2 • Ready in 12 minutes

1 tbsp sesame seeds

1 cucumber, spiralized and blotted on kitchen paper

100g baby kale, roughly chopped

60g pak choi, very finely shredded

½ red onion, very finely sliced

Large handful (20g) parsley, chopped

150g cooked chicken, shredded

For the dressing:

1 tbsp extra virgin olive oil

1 tsp sesame oil

Juice of 1 lime

1 tsp clear honey

2 tsp soy sauce

- Toast the sesame seeds in a dry frying pan for 2 minutes until lightly browned and fragrant.

- In a small bowl, mix together the olive oil, sesame oil, lime juice, honey and soy sauce to make the dressing.

- Place the cucumber, kale, pak choi, red onion and parsley in a large bowl and gently mix together. Pour over the dressing and mix again.

- Distribute the salad between two plates and top with the shredded chicken. Sprinkle over the sesame seeds just before serving.

Cucumber and Asparagus Salad with Prosciutto

249 calories

This is a fab salad for when asparagus is in season.

Serves 1 • Ready in 10 minutes

1 large egg, pricked
100g young asparagus, trimmed
10 cherry tomatoes, quartered
1 tsp extra virgin olive oil
1 tsp balsamic vinegar
½ cucumber, spiralized and blotted on kitchen paper
1 slice prosciutto or parma ham, cut into pieces
5g (1 tsp) parmesan cheese, finely grated
salt and freshly ground black pepper

- Bring a small saucepan of water to a fast boil. Slowly lower the egg into the water and cook for 7-8 minutes. Remove the egg from the water and peel under cold running water. Set aside.

- Lightly cook the asparagus by plunging into boiling water and boiling for 4–5 minutes, until just tender.

- Mix together the cherry tomatoes with the olive oil and balsamic vinegar.

- Put the cucumber noodles on a serving plate and arrange the asparagus on top. Pour the cherry tomatoes over. Next, add the prosciutto.

- Quarter the egg and add it to the pile. Finally, sprinkle on the Parmesan cheese and season generously.

Superfood Salad Bowl

443 calories

This delicious salad combines salmon with vegetables, nuts and seeds to get as much healthy goodness as you can in one bowl.

Serves 1 • Ready in 15 minutes

10g whole almonds

10g cashews

10g sunflower seeds

10g pomegranate seeds

1 small salmon fillet (100g), skinless and boneless

2 tsp soy sauce

½ tsp honey

¼ tsp ground ginger

5 florets (40g) of broccoli

Handful (40g) of sugar snap peas

½ small cucumber, spiralized and blotted on kitchen paper

1 fresh mint leaf, finely chopped (optional)

Small bunch (10g) of flat-leaf parsley, finely chopped (optional)

1 spring onion, chopped

- Place a small dry frying pan over a medium heat until toasty hot. Toss in the almonds, cashews and seeds. Dry fry for a few minutes, stirring frequently, until they release their aromas and start to brown. Remove from the pan and set aside.

- Cut the salmon in half lengthways and add to the still hot pan. Fry the salmon in its own oil for about 4 minutes each side, until just cooked through. Remove from the pan and set aside.

- Meanwhile, prepare the honey dressing for the salmon. In a shallow bowl, mix together the soy sauce, honey and ginger. As soon as the salmon is cool enough to handle roughly flake with your fingers into the dressing. Spoon the dressing over so that the salmon is fully covered. Leave to rest while you prepare the rest of the salad.

- Simmer the broccoli and sugar snap peas together for approximately 6 minutes until tender.

- Arrange the spiralized cucumber, herbs (if using) and spring onions on a serving plate or bowl. Add the broccoli and sugar snaps. Arrange the salmon over the top and sprinkle on the nuts and seeds. Finally drizzle over any remaining dressing.

Cucumber Egg Florentine

313 calories

A poached egg with hollandaise sauce is a perfect easy meal for one. I use a quick 'cheats' hollandaise here.

Serves 1 • Ready in 12 minutes

2 large eggs
1 tbsp thick mayonnaise
¼ tsp Dijon mustard
Juice of ½ lemon
1 tsp extra-virgin olive oil
Pinch of salt
Pinch of cayenne pepper
Pinch of turmeric (optional, for colour only)
½ cucumber, spiralized and blotted on kitchen paper
2 thick slices beef tomato
Pinch of paprika

- Fill a wide pan with 4–5cm water. Bring up to simmering point. The water should be just simmering with a few occasional bubbles.

- Crack the first egg on the side of the pan and then gently lower it into the water. Repeat with the second egg. Simmer for exactly 1 minute before turning the heat off and leaving the eggs to cook in the slowly cooling water for a further 10 minutes. This should ensure a cooked egg with a runny middle.

- Meanwhile prepare the mock hollandaise. Put the

mayonnaise, mustard, lemon juice, olive oil, salt, cayenne pepper and turmeric in a small bowl or jug and whisk together until smooth.

- Arrange the spiralized cucumber on a plate and add the tomato slices. Then, using a slotted spoon, carefully transfer the eggs to the top of each tomato slice. Pour over the hollandaise sauce and top with a pinch of paprika.

Oriental Salmon Fishcakes on Lime Noodles

455 calories

These elegant, oriental-style fishcakes are a bit different from the norm.

Serves 2 • Ready in 12 minutes

2 skinless salmon fillets (approximately 130g each), cut into chunks
2 spring onions, chopped
1 small egg, beaten
2 heaped tbsp plain flour
1 tbsp desiccated coconut
½ tsp nam pla fish sauce
Small handful of fresh coriander, roughly chopped
Juice of ½ lime
2 tbsp olive oil
1 cucumber, spiralized and blotted on kitchen paper
1 tsp walnut oil
Juice of half lime
1 tbsp soy sauce
Lime wedges, to serve

- Place the salmon in a food processor and pulse briefly. Add the spring onions, egg, gram flour, coconut, fish sauce, coriander and lime juice to the salmon and blitz again until roughly combined.

- Heat the oil in a heavy-based frying pan and when hot add tablespoons of the salmon mixture to the pan. Press down lightly on the top of the salmon to make them into patties no more than 1cm thick. Cook for 2–3 minutes each side and turn gently with a fish slice. Be careful as they can be delicate.

- Toss the spiralized cucumber with the walnut oil, lime juice and soy sauce. Serve the fishcakes on the noodles with a wedge of lime on the side.

Japanese-style Sake Prawn Salad

178 calories

A very healthy Japanese-style salad.

Serves 2 • Ready in 8 minutes

2 tbsp water
....
2 tbsp sake
....
pinch of salt
....
juice of 1 lime
....
½ tsp wasabi powder
....
2 tsp olive oil
....
1 garlic clove, peeled and crushed
....
2 spring onions, trimmed and sliced
....
250g raw king prawns, fresh or frozen
....
1 cucumber, spiralized and blotted on
kitchen paper
....

• In a small bowl, mix together the water, sake, salt, lime juice and wasabi powder.

• Heat the oil in a wide frying pan over a high heat. When hot, add the garlic and spring onions and fry lightly for 1–2 minutes. Tip in the prawns and cook for about 2 minutes (fresh) or 4 minutes (frozen), until they just start to turn pink.

• Tip in the sake mixture and bring up to a vigorous simmer. Cook for 2 minutes, stirring occasionally.

• When the prawns are cooked, serve on a bed of cucumber noodles with a little of the sauce from the pan drizzled over.

Tinned Salmon and Bean Salad

346 calories

This is a fantastic 'storecupboard' salad that can be on the table in 5 minutes. Although it serves two, I tend to make it just for me and refrigerate half. It keeps well in the fridge for up to two days and I think tastes even better the next day.

Serves 2 • Ready in 5 minutes

½ red onion, peeled and cut into half rings

1 tbsp extra virgin olive oil

juice of 1 lemon

1 × 200g can salmon

1 × 400g can mixed beans, rinsed and drained

salt and freshly ground black pepper

1 cucumber, spiralized and blotted on kitchen paper

- Place the sliced onion in a small microwaveable bowl. Add the olive oil and lemon juice. Cover the bowl with clingfilm and microwave on high for 2 minutes. Leave to rest, covered, for a further 2 minutes.

- In a larger bowl, mix together the salmon and mixed beans. Pour the softened onion, oil and lemon juice over and combine. Season with salt and pepper. It can be refrigerated at this stage if desired.

- Lightly toss through the spiralized cucumber before serving.

Paprika Chicken Noodles

286 calories

One of my favourite easy noodles, the chicken is very tender when quick fried in this way.

Serves 1 • Ready in 15 minutes

1 × 150g skinless chicken breast, cut into 4–5 slices

1 tsp plain flour

salt and freshly ground black pepper

½ tsp paprika

1 tsp olive oil

20g baby leaf spinach

½ cucumber, spiralized and blotted on kitchen paper

1 tbsp natural yogurt

1 tsp extra virgin olive oil

¼ tsp paprika

- Place the chicken in a bowl and sprinkle on the flour, salt and pepper and ½ teaspoon paprika. Use your hands to toss the chicken in the flour and make sure it is evenly covered.

- Heat the oil in a frying pan over a medium heat. When hot, add the chicken and fry for about 4-6 minutes on each side, depending on thickness.

- Meanwhile, arrange the spinach and cucumber noodles in a serving bowl. Combine the yogurt, extra virgin olive oil and ¼ teaspoon paprika in a small cup.

- Place the just cooked chicken on top of the salad and drizzle the yogurt dressing over.

Avocado and Bacon Salad

285 calories

Always a fab flavour combination!

Serves 1 • Ready in 15 minutes

15g streaky bacon, chopped (about 1 slice)

¼ red onion, finely sliced

½ red pepper, finely sliced

½ cucumber, spiralized and blotted on kitchen paper

20g young leaf spinach

½ ripe avocado, sliced

1 tsp extra virgin olive oil

juice of ½ lemon

salt and freshly ground black pepper

- Heat a small frying pan over a medium–high heat and fry the bacon until brown and crisp. Dry and cool on kitchen paper.

- Using the oil left in the pan from the bacon, reduce the heat a little and fry the onion and red pepper for 5–7 minutes until tender and golden.

- Place the cucumber noodles and spinach leaves in a wide bowl and mix through the onion and red pepper. Add the sliced avocado and drizzle with the olive oil and lemon juice. Season with salt and pepper and top with the crispy bacon.

Lime Salsa Prawns

222 calories

Serves 1 • Ready in 10 minutes

1 medium tomato, diced

¼ red onion, peeled and finely diced

½ small red chilli, deseeded and finely chopped

1 tsp olive oil

juice of 1 lime

salt and freshly ground black pepper

150g cooked prawns

handful of fresh coriander, chopped

1 little Gem lettuce, roughly chopped

½ cucumber, spiralized and blotted on kitchen paper

- Place the tomato, red onion and chilli in a small bowl and add the oil, lime juice and salt and pepper. Leave to mellow for 5 minutes.
- Combine the prawns and coriander in a bowl. Then mix in the marinated tomato and onion.
- Mix the lettuce and spiralized cucumber on a serving plate and scoop the prawns and salsa over.

Creamy Cucumber Noodles with Baked Salmon

316 calories

Quick and easy baked salmon with a delicious creamy dressing.

Serves 1 • Ready in 20 minutes

1 skinless salmon fillet, about 130g

1 tsp low-fat mayonnaise

1 tbsp natural yogurt

1 tbsp rice wine vinegar

2 fresh mint leaves, finely chopped

salt and freshly ground black pepper

½ cucumber, spiralized and blotted on kitchen paper

2 radishes, thinly sliced

2 spring onions, trimmed and sliced

- Preheat the oven to 200C/180C fan.

- Place the salmon fillet on a baking tray and bake in the oven for 16–18 minutes until just cooked through. Remove from the oven and set aside – the salmon is equally nice hot or cold in the salad.

- In a small bowl, mix the mayonnaise, yogurt, vinegar, mint and salt and pepper together and leave to stand for at least 5 minutes to allow the flavours to develop.

- Arrange the spiralized cucumber on a serving plate and top with the radishes, cucumber and spring onions. Gently stir in half the dressing. Flake the salmon over the top and drizzle the remaining dressing over.

Smoked Mackerel and Lentils

407 calories

Smoked mackerel goes beautifully with the cucumber noodles.

Serves 1 • Ready in 5 minutes

½ cucumber, spiralized and blotted on kitchen paper
....
10 cherry tomatoes, halved
....
50g ready-to-eat puy lentils
....
juice of ½ lemon, plus an extra squeeze
....
1 tsp extra virgin olive oil
....
salt and freshly ground black pepper
....
80g smoked mackerel fillets
....

- Place the spiralized cucumber in a serving bowl and add the cherry tomatoes and lentils.

- Mix the lemon juice, olive oil and salt and pepper in a small bowl. Pour over the salad and toss lightly. Flake the mackerel over the top and squeeze over a little extra lemon juice before serving.

Garlic Butter Chicken

319 calories

A very flavoursome chicken salad.

Serves 2 • Ready in 15 minutes

2 cloves garlic, peeled and crushed
1 tbsp extra virgin olive oil
½ tsp dried oregano/mixed herbs
Freshly ground black pepper
20g butter, at room temperature
2 × 150g skinless chicken breast fillets, cut into strips
1 cucumber, spiralized and blotted on kitchen paper
50g rocket leaves
1 tsp white wine vinegar

- In a small bowl, combine the garlic, olive oil, dried herbs and black pepper. Set aside 1 teaspoon of the mixture to dress the salad. Add the butter to the bowl and mix until you have a smooth paste.

- Add the garlic butter to the chicken strips and use your hands to rub the butter all over the chicken pieces. Rest the chicken in the butter for 5-10 minutes if possible.

- Heat a wide frying pan to a medium heat and when hot toss in the chicken strips. Cook for 10–12 minutes until browned and fully cooked, stirring regularly. Remove from the pan. The chicken can be used hot or cold in the salad.

- Arrange the spiralized cucumber and rocket leaves

over two serving plates. Add the white wine vinegar to the set aside garlic oil and pour over the two salads. Top with the cooked chicken.

Pomegranate, Feta and Walnut Salad

395 calories

A totally delicious combination of flavours.

Serves 1 • Ready in 5 minutes

½ cucumber, spiralized and blotted on kitchen paper

50g ready-to-eat or cooked puy lentils

30g feta cheese, cut into cubes

20g pomegranate seeds

20g walnuts, halved

For the dressing:

1 tbsp Greek yogurt

1 tsp rice vinegar

Pinch of sugar

1 tsp extra virgin olive oil

2 leaves mint, finely chopped

- Combine the Greek yogurt, rice vinegar, sugar, extra virgin olive oil and chopped mint in a small bowl.
- Arrange the spiralized cucumber and lentils on a serving dish. Top with the feta, pomegranate and walnuts. Drizzle the dressing over the top and serve.

OTHER SPIRALIZER RECIPES

Although courgettes, carrots and cucumbers are some of the most popular vegetables to spiralize you don't need to stop there. Any firm and solid vegetable or fruit should spiralize pretty well. Parsnip, cabbage, onion and apple can all be spiralized beautifully.

• • •

Chicken Caesar Salad with Carrot Noodles

Roasted Red Onion Pasta

Quick Vegetable Stir-Fry with Blackbean Sauce

Spiralized Cabbage with Stilton

Beef and Celeriac Gratin

Parsnip and Leek Frittata

Butternut Squash Crumble

Celeriac Remoulade with Smoked Trout

Roasted Butternut Squash Spirals with Fried Halloumi

Thai Chicken Salad

Oven-baked Onion Bhajis

Stir-fry Pork with Red Cabbage and Apple

Seared Beef with Vegetable Coleslaw

Caramelized Apples with Ice Cream

Apple Spaghetti and Ginger Crunch

Chicken Caesar Salad with Carrot Noodles

430 calories

This is an easy salad to rustle up if you have some leftover cooked chicken.

Serves 1 • Ready in 5 minutes

Handful (10g) of pine nuts
....

2 tbsp French-style mayonnaise
....

1 tsp white wine vinegar
....

½ tsp Worcestershire sauce
....

1 heaped tsp capers, crushed
....

Freshly ground black pepper
....

100g cooked chicken breast, skin removed, sliced
....

1 large (or 2 small carrots), peeled and spiralized
....

4 large black olives
....

10g Parmesan cheese, finely grated
....

- Heat a small dry frying pan over a medium/high heat. Toss in the pine nuts and cook for about 2 minutes, gently shaking the pan at intervals to make sure they're toasted all over. Transfer to a plate to cool.

- Combine the mayonnaise, vinegar, Worcestershire sauce, crushed capers and freshly ground black pepper in a bowl. Add the sliced chicken and mix lightly.

- Arrange the carrot in a wide bowl and add the dressed chicken. Top with the black olives, Parmesan and toasted pine nuts.

Roasted Red Onion Pasta

207 calories

A great little 'bung it all in a baking dish and forget about it' kinda recipe.

Serves 2 • Ready in 30 minutes

2 red onions, peeled and quartered
4 cloves garlic, unpeeled
2 sprigs thyme (or 1 tsp dried thyme)
250g cherry tomatoes, halved
Salt and freshly ground black pepper
1 tbsp olive oil
1 tsp English mustard
1 tsp extra virgin olive oil
1 tbsp red wine vinegar
1 tsp honey

- Preheat the oven to 220C/200C fan.

- Pass the red onion through the spiralizer or use a julienne peeler. You should get short delicate curls of 'pasta'.

- Place the red onion in a bowl and add the garlic cloves, thyme and cherry tomatoes. Season generously with salt and pepper and pour over the oil. Use your hands to toss the oil through the vegetables. Transfer to a roasting tin and cook in the oven for 20-25 minutes.

- Remove from the oven and with a fork, crush the garlic cloves. Remove any excess skin and mix together.

- In a small bowl, combine the mustard, extra virgin olive oil, red wine vinegar and honey. Toss through the onion pasta and serve.

Quick Vegetable Stir-Fry with Blackbean Sauce

316 calories

A tasty and easy vegetarian dinner.

Serves 2 • Ready in 10 minutes

250g firm tofu, cut into large cubes
100g cooked black beans, rinsed and drained
2 heaped tsp (30g) blackcurrant jam
½ tsp ground ginger
1 tbsp dark soy sauce
1 tsp cornflour
salt and freshly ground black pepper
1 tbsp olive oil
¼ small celeriac, peeled and spiralized
¼ white cabbage, stalk removed, cored and spiralized
2 carrots, peeled and spiralized
100g curly kale, stalks removed and cut thinly

- Spread the tofu out on a plate covered in kitchen paper. Cover with kitchen paper and set aside.

- Place the blackbeans, blackcurrant jam, ginger, soy sauce and cornflour into a food processor and blend until smooth.

- Season the tofu generously with the salt and pepper. Heat the oil in a wide frying pan or wok. On a high heat, stir-fry the tofu until golden brown all over. Remove from the pan with a slotted spoon and set aside. Add the celeriac, cabbage, carrot and kale to the pan and stir-fry for 5-6 minutes.

- Reduce the heat to medium-low and return the tofu to the pan. Add the black-bean sauce and warm through for 2 minutes before serving.

Spiralized Cabbage with Stilton

237 calories

Serves 2 • Ready in 20 minutes

1 tsp olive oil

1 leek, trimmed and sliced

1 small potato (100g), peeled and diced

¼ to ½ savoy cabbage, outer leaves
removed and spiralized

1 tbsp sherry

1 tbsp double cream

50g stilton, crumbled

freshly ground black pepper

Heat the oil in a large lidded pan and gently fry the leeks, potato and cabbage for 5 minutes. Then add 2-3 tbsp water, put the lid on the pan and steam for a further 5-10 minutes or until tender.

Add the sherry and cream and lightly simmer for a minute. Stir in the Stilton and freshly ground black pepper before serving.

Beef and Celeriac Gratin

310 calories

This recipe is made in two stages. First you make a wine sauce and marinate the beef in the sauce overnight before assembling the pie. I promise you it is well worth the effort.

Serves 4 • Ready in 2 hours + overnight marinating

1 tsp olive oil

1 large onion, peeled and finely chopped

1 celery stick, trimmed and finely chopped

1 garlic clove, peeled and finely chopped

1 bay leaf

200ml red wine

400g lean casserole beef steak

1 tbsp plain flour

250g button mushrooms

1 tsp English mustard

500ml beef stock (fresh or made from 1 cube)

1 medium celeriac (about 800g)

salt and freshly ground black pepper

50g wholemeal breadcrumbs

1 tbsp extra virgin olive oil

• Heat the oil in a frying pan over a medium heat. Add the onion and celery and fry for 5 minutes. Add the garlic, bay leaf and red wine and bring to the boil. Reduce the heat and simmer for 10 minutes. Leave to cool.

- Place the beef in a wide bowl and pour the wine mixture over. Cover and refrigerate overnight or for at least 4 hours.
- Preheat the oven to 180C/160C fan.
- Put the marinated beef in the base of a large baking dish, together with the marinade. Sprinkle over the flour, then add the mushrooms.
- Stir the mustard into the beef stock and pour over the mushrooms. You want the mushrooms to be just covered but not swimming in the stock. Bake in the oven for 90 minutes.
- Meanwhile, prepare the celeriac. Half fill a large saucepan with cold salted water. Use a knife to top and tail the celeriac before trimming off the skin. Quarter the celeriac lengthways. Spiralize the celeriac and add to the cold water. Bring to the boil, and simmer for 5 minutes until just tender. Drain the celeriac and leave to cool.
- Remove the baking dish from the oven and layer half the celeriac on top, pushing the celeriac down gently into the beef sauce. Then add a final layer of celeriac and sprinkle on the breadcrumbs. Season with salt and pepper and drizzle over the extra virgin olive oil.
- Bake in the oven uncovered for 30–40 minutes until golden.

Parsnip and Leek Frittata

297 calories

This is as good cold as hot, so keep the second half for your lunchbox tomorrow.

Serves 2 • Ready in 30 minutes

2 tsp olive oil

2 leeks, trimmed and chopped

2 medium parsnips, about 80g each, peeled and spiralized

3 large eggs

½ tsp English mustard

30g Pecorino cheese, finely grated

freshly ground black pepper

- In a lidded frying pan heat 1 tsp of oil over a medium–high heat. Toss in the leeks and spiralized parsnips and stir-fry for 2 minutes. Reduce the heat, add 2 tablespoons water and put the lid on. Sweat the leeks and parsnips for 10 minutes or until tender. Leave to cool.

- Put the eggs and mustard in a bowl and whisk thoroughly with a fork. Stir in half the grated cheese and cooled vegetables.

- Preheat the grill to a medium setting.

- Choose a frying pan with a metal handle that can go under the grill. Wipe with kitchen paper dipped in the remaining oil. Heat over a medium–high heat and, when hot, add the egg mixture. Roll the pan around so the egg covers the base of the pan evenly. Immediately turn the heat to the lowest setting and cook, uncovered, for about 10 minutes or until the base and sides are firm.

- Sprinkle over the black pepper and remaining cheese. Put the pan under the grill for another 5–10 minutes until the top is firm and golden.

- Turn out onto a plate. Serve immediately or leave to cool and serve in wedges.

Butternut Squash Crumble

321 calories

This is a super healthy and filling vegetarian meal.

Serves 4 • Ready in 1 hour 30 minutes

2 tbsp olive oil

1 large onion, peeled and chopped

2 garlic cloves, peeled and sliced

1 red chilli, deseeded and chopped

300ml white wine

500ml vegetable stock (fresh or made with one cube)

1 bay leaf

1 tsp dried thyme

800g butternut squash (about 1 large), peeled, deseeded and spiralized

1 × 400g can butterbeans

50g wholemeal breadcrumbs

25g porridge oats

25g cashews, roughly chopped

handful of fresh parsley, chopped

Salt and freshly ground black pepper

- Heat 1 tablespoon of oil in a large pan, add the onion and fry gently for 8 minutes. Add the garlic and chilli and fry for a further 2 minutes.

- Stir in the white wine, vegetable stock, bay leaf and thyme. Bring to the boil, then reduce the heat to medium–low and simmer, uncovered, for 20 minutes.

- Add the butternut squash and cook for a further

10 minutes. Stir in the butter beans including their soaking liquor.

- Preheat the oven 180C/160C fan.

- Mix the breadcrumbs, oats, chopped cashews, parsley and the remaining tablespoon of oil together.

- Transfer the vegetable sauce to a suitable casserole dish and sprinkle on the crumble topping. Season liberally with salt and pepper. Bake in the oven for 30 minutes or until the crumble is golden and crisp.

Celeriac Remoulade with Smoked Trout

220 calories

Think of this as a tangy celeriac coleslaw.

Serves 1 • Ready in 15 minutes

¼ small celeriac, about 150g peeled weight
50g rocket
1 tbsp mayonnaise
1 tbsp natural yogurt
1 tbsp capers, chopped
juice ½ lemon
1 gherkin or 2 cornichons, chopped
salt and freshly ground black pepper
60g smoked trout, flaked
lemon wedge, to serve

- Peel the celeriac and spiralize. Combine the celeriac with the rocket.

- In a small bowl, mix together the mayonnaise, yogurt, capers, lemon juice and chopped gherkin. Season with salt and pepper.

- Pour the dressing over the celeriac and mix until the celeriac and rocket are both covered.

- Arrange the smoked trout over the top and serve with a lemon wedge.

Roasted Butternut Squash Spirals with Fried Halloumi

329 calories

A simple and filling dinner.

Serves 1 • Ready in 5 minutes

½ tsp cumin seeds
2 tsp olive oil
40g halloumi, cut into cubes
½ tsp chilli flakes
Freshly ground black pepper
200g butternut squash (peeled weight), spiralized or julienned
10g butter
Juice of 1 lime
Fresh coriander leaves (optional)

- In a wide pan, dry fry the cumin seeds for a minute or two. Then add the olive oil and fry the halloumi until browned all over. Add the chilli flakes, black pepper and butternut squash. Fry for 2-4 minutes, or until the squash starts to brown.

- Add the butter and stir through when melted. Finally add the lime juice and coriander leaves (if using). Stir and serve immediately.

Thai Chicken Salad

283 calories

Lots of spiralizing here – the carrots, cucumber, cabbage and red onion can all be spiralized.

Serves 2 • Ready in 10 minutes

1 large carrot, peeled and spiralized

½ cucumber, peeled and spiralized

¼ white cabbage, core removed and spiralized

¼ red onion, spiralized

Handful fresh coriander leaves, roughly chopped

200g cooked chicken breast, thinly sliced

30g cashews, roughly chopped

For the dressing:

1 tbsp Thai fish sauce

1 tbsp mirin or cooking sherry

1 tsp chilli flakes

1 tsp palm sugar or soft brown sugar

½ tsp ground ginger

1 tbsp rice vinegar

Juice of half a lime

- Spiralize all the vegetables and mix together in a large bowl with the coriander leaves.
- Prepare the dressing by combining the fish sauce, mirin, chilli flakes, palm sugar, ground ginger, rice vinegar and lime juice in a small bowl. Stir until well combined. Pour half the dressing over the vegetables and stir well.

- Distribute the salad between two plates and arrange the chicken over. Pour over the remains of the dressing and finally top with cashews.

Oven-baked Onion Bhajis

45 calories per bhaji

By using a spiralizer to make easy work of the onions, these onion bhajis are a breeze.

Makes 8 bhajis • Ready in 35 minutes

1 tbsp olive oil
2 white onions, peeled and spiralized
1 tsp granulated sugar
1 thumb fresh ginger, peeled and grated
½ tsp ground cumin
1 tsp mild chilli powder
½ tsp chilli flakes
1 tsp salt
2 tbsp gram (chickpea) flour

- Heat the oil in a lidded pan on a high heat. Add the white onions and sugar, stir and sizzle for 2 minutes before turning the heat down to low, placing the lid on the pan and cooking slowly for 10-15 minutes until the onions are soft and browned. Leave to cool.
- Preheat the oven to 220C/200C fan.
- In a large bowl, mix the cooked onions, ginger, cumin, chilli powder, chilli flakes, salt and gram flour. Use a dessert spoon to drop balls of the mix onto a large baking tray. Bake in the oven for 20 minutes, or until crispy.

Stir-fry Pork with Red Cabbage and Apple

394 calories

The sweet cabbage and apple goes beautifully with the salted pork.

Serves 2 • Ready in 1 hour

1 tsp olive oil
1 red onion, peeled and spiralized
1 garlic clove, peeled and chopped
1 tbsp caraway seeds (optional)
½ medium red cabbage (about 400g), quartered, cored and spiralized
2 apples, peeled, cored and spiralized
juice and zest of ½ lemon
1 tsp balsamic vinegar
salt and freshly ground black pepper
1 tsp olive oil
1 tsp walnut oil
2 lean pork steaks (approx. 125g each), cut into strips
1 tbsp soy sauce

- Heat the olive oil in a large lidded saucepan over a medium heat and fry the onion for 5 minutes until soft and lightly caramelized. Add the garlic and caraway seeds and cook for 30 seconds or until the seeds start to pop.

- Add the cabbage, apple, lemon juice and balsamic vinegar, together with 100ml water and a generous seasoning of salt and pepper. Put the lid on, reduce the heat to low and cook for 45 minutes or until tender. Stir and check the water levels once or twice during cooking. If there's still a little water left in the pan at the end of the cooking time, remove the lid and cook for another 5 minutes. The red cabbage can also be slow cooked in a low oven or slow cooker on low for 4–6 hours.

- While the cabbage is cooking, toss the strips of pork with the oils and soy sauce. Heat a frying pan on a medium-high heat. Toss in the pork strips and fry until browned all over and cooked through. Serve over the cooked cabbage.

Seared Beef with Vegetable Coleslaw

484 calories

Spiralizers were made for coleslaw. You could also add fennel, radishes or beetroot to the vegetable mix.

Serves 2 • Ready in 20 minutes

1 carrot, peeled and spiralized
¼ celeriac, peeled and spiralized
¼ white cabbage, outer leaves removed, cored and spiralized
1 shallot, peeled and sliced
Juice of half a lemon
1 tbsp extra virgin olive oil
100g natural yogurt
2 tsp English mustard
Salt and freshly ground black pepper
2 small beef fillet steaks (approx. 125g each)
1 tsp olive oil

- Mix the carrot, celeriac, cabbage and shallot in a large bowl. In a separate bowl, mix the lemon juice, extra virgin olive oil, yogurt and English mustard. Combine with the veg and season generously with salt and pepper.

- Prepare the beef steaks by rubbing with the olive oil and a little salt and pepper. Heat a pan to a very high heat and cook for 2-6 minutes each side. The cooking time will depend on (a) how cooked you like your meat and (b) how thick the steaks are.

- Serve the steaks next to a generous dollop of the coleslaw.

Caramelized Apples with Ice Cream

219 calories (without ice cream)

Spiralized apples are delicious. Don't overcook or they could become mushy.

Serves 2 • Ready in 10 minutes

Juice of 1 lemon
4 crisp apples
20g butter
2 tbsp granulated sugar
Good quality vanilla ice cream to serve

- First prepare a bowl for the spiralized apples. The apples will start turning brown as soon as the flesh is exposed to air so be prepared. Take a large bowl and half fill with cold water. Add the lemon juice.

- Next prepare the apples one at a time. First peel, quarter and core the apple. Then spiralize the apple quarters straight into the water. Push down so that no apple is exposed.

- Melt the butter with the sugar over a low-medium heat until sugar dissolves and the mixture is just bubbly. Pull handfuls of the apple out of the water, shake off any excess water and add to the pan. Stir in quickly. Repeat until all the apples are in the pan. Now turn up the heat a little and stir constantly for 5-8 minutes until the apples are soft and golden.

- Serve hot or cold over the ice cream.

Apple Spaghetti and Ginger Crunch

265 calories

This is a very special crumble.

Serves 4 • Ready in 45 minutes

juice of 1 lemon

4 crisp eating apples

75g porridge oats

1 tbsp flaked almonds, lightly crushed

2 tbsp runny honey

40g butter

1 tbsp crystallized ginger, chopped

1 tbsp demerara sugar

- Preheat the oven to 180C/160C fan.

- Prepare a bowl for the apple. Half fill a large bowl with cold water and add the lemon juice. Peel, quarter and core the apples and spiralize straight into the prepared bowl. Leave submerged under the water to prevent discolouration.

- Mix the oats and almonds in a mixing bowl. Melt the honey and butter together in the microwave or small saucepan until just combined (but not bubbling) and pour over the oat mixture. Stir well.

- Take a medium baking dish. Pull handfuls of the apple out of the water, lightly shake and arrange over the base of the dish. Distribute the crystallized ginger over. Spoon over the oat crunch and finally add the demerara sugar. Bake in the oven for 30–40 minutes until crisped and lightly golden.

INDEX

10114458R00086

Printed in Germany
by Amazon Distribution
GmbH, Leipzig